OXFORD MEDICAL PUBLICATIONS

Epidemiology in General Practice

OXFORD GENERAL PRACTICE SERIES

2. Geriatric problems in general practice
   G. Wilcock, J. A. M. Gray, and P. M. M. Pritchard
3. Preventive medicine in general practice
   edited by J. A. M. Gray and G. H. Fowler
5. Locomotor disability in general practice
   edited by M. I. V. Jayson and R. Million
6. The consultation: an approach to learning and teaching
   D. Pendleton, P. Tate, P. Havelock, and T. P. C. Schofield
7. Continuing care: the management of chronic disease
   edited by J. C. Hasler and T. P. C. Schofield
8. Management in general practice
   P. M. M. Pritchard, K. B. Low, and M. Whalen
9. Modern obstetrics in general practice
   edited by G. N. Marsh
10. Terminal care at home
    edited by R. Spilling
11. Rheumatology for general practitioners
    H. L. F. Currey and S. Hull
12. Women's problems in general practice
    (Second edition)
    edited by Ann McPherson
13. Paediatric problems in general practice
    (Second edition)
    M. Modell and R. H. Boyd
14. Epidemiology in general practice
    edited by David Morrell

Epidemiology in General Practice

Oxford General Practice Series 14

Edited by

DAVID MORRELL
Wolfson Professor of General Practice,
The United Medical and Dental Schools of
Guy's and St. Thomas's Hospitals

OXFORD NEW YORK TORONTO MELBOURNE
OXFORD UNIVERSITY PRESS
1988

Oxford University Press, Walton Street, Oxford OX2 6DP
Oxford New York Toronto
Delhi Bombay Calcutta Madras Karachi
Petaling Jaya Singapore Hong Kong Tokyo
Nairobi Dar es Salaam Cape Town
Melbourne Auckland
and associated companies in
Berlin Ibadan

Oxford is a trade mark of Oxford University Press

Published in the United States
by Oxford University Press, New York

British Library Cataloguing in Publication Data
Epidemiology in general practice.
1. Man. Diseases. Epidemiology.
Methodology
I. Morrell, David
614.4
ISBN 0-19-261603-X

Library of Congress Cataloging in Publication Data
Epidemiology in general practice.
(Oxford general practice series; 14) (Oxford medical publications)
1. Family medicine. 2. Epidemiology. I. Morrell, David Cameron. II. Series: Oxford general practice series; no. 14. III. Series: Oxford medical publications. [DNLM: 1. Epidemiologic Methods. 2. Epidemiology. 3. Family Practice. W1 OX55 no. 14/W 89 E64]
R729.5.G4E64 1988 614.4 88-15115
ISBN 0-19-261603-X (pbk.)

Typeset by Cotswold Typesetting Ltd., Gloucester
Printed in Great Britain
at the University Printing House, Oxford
by David Stanford
Printer to the University

Foreword

BY WALTER HOLLAND, MD, FRCP, FRCGP, FFCM

As an epidemiologist I have always been surprised at how little use general practitioners make of the opportunities that present themselves for the investigation of disease in the surgery. The general practitioner is the first contact for any individual with a symptom and is often able to study families and populations. He frequently follows individuals from the onset of disease until death and holds a vantage point from which to judge the effectiveness of a wide spectrum of medical procedures. General practitioners also have great opportunities to prevent illness and disability, and as gate-keepers to the hospital they can allocate resources to those in greatest need. It is rare, however, to observe the general practice as the setting for the scientific study of the natural history of disease or the effectiveness of health care.

None the less, general practitioners have made significant contributions. The association between thalidomide and congenital malformations was first recognized by a general practitioner, McBride (1961). Knowledge of the spread and infectiousness of jaundice and the distinction between chicken pox and shingles stems from the work of Pickles (1939).

In the past the chief medical concern was for acute infectious diseases (Budd 1873; Pickles 1939) whose signs and symptoms are relatively easy to detect. The general practitioner performed an important research function if his observations were diligent and his records well kept. However, the considerable increase in the incidence of chronic disease has necessitated a sophistication of recording methods and the need to elicit reliable information about patient life-style.

Professor Morrell's department is unique as a Department of General Practice in the care taken with data that are collected. In the execution of studies, the reliability and validity of observations are always questioned. Thus the accuracy with which clerks record attendance at the surgery is checked, and if it is found wanting appropriate remedial action is taken. Methods of recording diagnoses and even symptoms accurately and repeatedly have been refined. This book provides a superb introduction to the concepts and methods that the general practitioner should use if conducting epidemiological research in the general practice setting, and illustrates particularly well the care that should be taken in collecting data and the measurements required to investigate complex issues such as the epidemiology of chronic diseases and psychiatric disorders.

December 1987

REFERENCES

Budd, W. (1873). *Typhoid fever*. London.
McBride, W. G. (1961). Thalidomide and congenital abnormalities. *Lancet* **ii,** 1358.
Pickles, W. N. (1939). *Epidemiology in general practice*. John Wright, Bristol.

Preface

Epidemiology is a scientific method which defines and measures events occurring in communities. It analyses and interprets these events in order to identify the relationships between them so as to explain the causes and outcome of illness, disease, and disability. This is a rather complicated way of saying that epidemiology has been used to identify the causes and outcomes of such common diseases and disabilities as chronic bronchitis, carcinoma of the lung, and stroke, or at a more basic level that it was used to identify the 'Broad Street pump' as the source of a major epidemic of cholera in London.

Such large community studies may seem remote from the day-to-day problems of doctors working in general practice, but the methods used are very relevant to solving many of these problems. The decision-making in general practice is concerned with an understanding of the incidence, prevalence, and natural history of symptoms of illness and disease. It is also concerned with the factors which influence individuals experiencing illness to consult a doctor. The interpretation of symptoms presenting in general practice and the use of diagnostic skills and investigations is largely governed by the knowledge of the probability of disease when common symptoms are presented and the sensitivity and specificity of the diagnostic procedures undertaken.

This book considers some of the problems experienced in a day or a year in the life of a general practitioner and indicates the ways in which epidemiological methods may be used to solve these problems. It is designed to encourage a critical approach, not just to the day-to-day problems but also to the information which medical journals and drug companies constantly direct at the general practitioner. It will help him to differentiate that which makes a real advance in knowledge and management and that which must be treated with healthy scepticism.

Epidemiology is not perhaps a word which warms the heart of the average general practitioner. It is, however, whether he likes it or not, the scientific method on which many of his decisions are made. This book is designed to help general practitioners respond more rationally and less negatively to a scientific method which demands discipline, numeracy, and logic, from which some enter general practice to escape but which many in due course realize is crucial to the provision of effective general practitioner care.

All the authors who have contributed to this book are general practitioners actively engaged in providing clinical care. It is from the problems which they encounter in their practices that they have developed their interests in epidemiology. It is hoped that their interest and enthusiasm will be as contagious as the water from the 'Broad Street pump'.

This book could not have been written without advice and encouragement from a large number of people. I would like to express my special thanks to Dr Peter Burney for his advice both on the epidemiological content of the book and on its general design. Mrs Carmel Stephenson has typed repeated drafts of the chapters with her usual diligence, patience, and good humour, without which the work would never have been completed. I am grateful to Mrs Margaret Neill for the line-drawings. Finally I thank my wife for her tolerance and encouragement.

London D.M.
1988

Contents

Contributors

David Morrell, OBE, KSG, MB, BS, FRCP, FRCGP, FFCM, DRCOG
Wolfson Professor of General Practice, The United Medical and Dental Schools of Guy's and St. Thomas's Hospitals.

Brian Jarman, MA, PHD, MRCP, FRCGP
Professor of Primary Health Care, St. Mary's Hospital Medical School.

Leone Ridsdale, BA, MSC(ECON), FRCPC, MRCGP
Senior Lecturer in General Practice, The United Medical and Dental Schools of Guy's and St. Thomas's Hospitals.

Martin Roland, MA, MRCP, MRCGP, DRCOG
Director of Studies in General Practice, Cambridge University School of Clinical Medicine.

Deborah Sharp, MA, BM, BCH, MRCGP, DRCOG
Lecturer in General Practice, The United Medical and Dental Schools of Guy's and St. Thomas's Hospitals.

Mike D'Souza, MD, FFCM, MRCGP
General Practitioner, Kingston, Surrey.

Christopher Watkins, PHD, FRCGP
Reader in General Practice, The United Medical and Dental Schools of Guy's and St. Thomas's Hospitals.

1 A day in the life of a general practitioner

David Morrell

Dr Preston had been a principal in the practice for six months. He found Wincampton a congenial town in which to live with his wife and two children and the population of 20 000 with the outlying villages provided plenty of work for the two group practices of four partners. On a mild September day with the leaves slowly turning to their autumn hues and the children reluctantly returning to school to cross-infect each other after their summer holidays, he started his morning surgery. He looked at the list of appointments booked at the statutory 6.66 minutes per patient and wondered, as he had often done, how he would get through by 11 o'clock when he was expected to finish and discuss with his partners, over a cup of coffee, the allocation of home visits. He could never understand how general practitioners had decided that 6.66 minutes was the appropriate time to allocate to consultations. He knew that at least four patients would attend without appointments and with what they described as emergency needs and they would be slotted in between the booked appointments. He just hoped that there would be an equal number of defaulters.

He sometimes wondered if the appointment system was worth all the work put into it because it seemed inevitable that some patients who had booked appointments would be kept waiting 15–20 minutes, and this seemed unfair when it was caused by patients requesting emergency consultations. It seemed very difficult to relate the services provided by the practice to the patients' demands for care and still more difficult to relate these demands to their real need for medical care. The more time the practice provided for consultations the more the demand increased and yet it was difficult to know how to control the demand short of turning patients away, and who should make this decision, the receptionists or the doctors? At 9 o'clock in the morning the problem seemed insoluble and he settled into his surgery consultations.

The first patient was aged 50. He had been started on treatment for hypertension identified at a routine pre-employment medical examination ten years before. He took methyldopa 250 mg four times daily and visited the practice at two-monthly intervals. His blood pressure was 140/90 and had been at this sort of level for the last twelve months. Dr Preston wondered if methyldopa was still the treatment of choice. He remembered a list of unpleasant side-effects attributed to this drug and recognized the benefits of beta blockers, but the patient seemed happy and he decided to let 'sleeping dogs lie'. He wondered if the patient really needed to be seen every two months or if three or six months would be more appropriate intervals, but he did not change the routine which had been established.

The second patient also suffered from hypertension and was about the same age. She was at least five stone overweight and her blood pressure was 160/90 (Fig. 1.1). She had been committed to a drug regime of beta blocker and diuretic on the basis of one blood pressure record of 170/105. He wondered if this was not normal for a patient with this degree of obesity. He could remember vaguely that arm circumference affected the measurement of blood pressure. As he reflected on the concept of normality with reference to this patient, he realized that her main problem was not her hypertension but her obesity. He decided to broach this subject and was somewhat dismayed when the patient assured him she scarcely ate anything all day. As he began to explore this area of her life she progressively became more aggressive and he felt progressively more impotent and increasingly angry. He finally repeated her prescription.

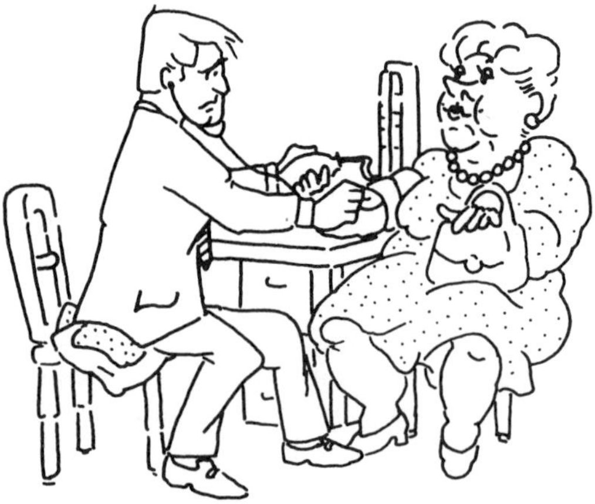

Fig. 1.1.

The next patient was 75 years old. She complained of increasing shortness of breath over a period of six months and increasing swelling of her ankles. She apologized for bothering him because she knew he was so busy, but she now found it impossible to climb the stairs to her flat. She was in gross cardiac failure. Dr Preston felt elated that he could prescribe drugs which would relieve her symptoms. At the same time he felt depressed that she should have tolerated this degree of disability for so long without seeking care. How many more patients like this were living in his community and struggling with increasing disability and failing to consult because 'he was so busy'? She had accepted cardiac failure as normal at her age and tried to live with it. Dr Preston wondered how this fitted with his concept of normality.

Two quick consultations followed with children. It was now 9.30a.m. on the first day of term. Dr Preston felt their mothers expected him to have some secret remedy for their coryza. He resisted the temptation to tell them about his previous patient who tolerated gross heart failure because he was so busy, and contented himself with reassuring them that they had at their disposal all the common remedies for the common cold and did not need a doctor's prescription.

The next patient was a 19-year-old mother with a 16-month-old child with a cough. The child was clearly not ill, and as the mother sat down the child jumped off her lap and proceeded to attack the pedal bin in the corner of the surgery (Fig. 1.2). The mother complained that he had a terrible cough which had disturbed her own and her husband's sleep. At first sight the child was healthy, apart from mild coryza, and further examination confirmed this. The consultation seemed totally inappropriate. Dr Preston had learned about this situation as a trainee and asked the patient the simple question 'why have you consulted me?' This brought an outpouring of abuse from the patient about her mother-in-law who said she was not fit to bring up a baby and about her husband, a long-distance lorry driver, who was always away from home. The diagnosis was coryza, but what did this say about the problems of this teenage mother and the complexity of their situation?

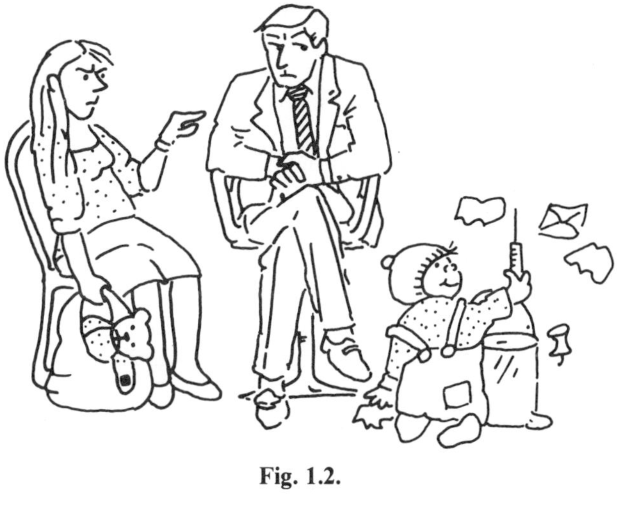

Fig. 1.2.

The next patient had seven children. She was sorry to bother the doctor but her three-year-old was having some difficulty in breathing. Dr Preston observed at once that the child looked pale, was quiet, and breathing with some difficulty. This child was clearly ill and he arranged an immediate admission to hospital. He reflected how important is an understanding of social factors and human behaviour in evaluating patients' requests for care.

Patient number eight had been seen a week previously complaining of dysuria and frequency of micturition. Dr Preston had sent a specimen of urine to the laboratory for microbiological examination and the report revealed no significant bacteriuria. While awaiting the report he had prescribed some antibiotics. The patient said at this consultation that she was now symptom-free. He asked himself what he had treated and what he had cured. It was clearly not a urinary tract infection defined in microbiological terms.

The next patient told him that her colitis was no better despite his treatment. It was clear from her record that full investigations of her upper and lower bowel had revealed no abnormalities. She was aged 35 and despite her efforts had not really succeeded in her ambitions in the Civil Service. What was the diagnosis and how could Dr Preston respond to satisfy her needs?

It was now 10 o'clock and Dr Preston was half-way through his morning surgery. He sat back in his chair and reflected on the last four patients. The first presented a symptom which clearly did not reflect her problems. The second case presented an acutely ill child who had not been brought to the doctor more expeditiously either because the mother was so busy with her brood or because she did not want to bother the doctor. The third had presented a clear-cut clinical syndrome which investigations had not supported. The fourth had presented a label of illness not supported by investigations and not responding to therapeutic endeavours. He was acutely conscious that this practice was part of the National Morbidity Survey in general practice organized by the Royal College of General Practitioners and the Office of Population Censuses and Surveys. For each of these consultations he had to record a diagnosis. He wondered what diagnosis he should record, and wondered even more about his patients' needs.

His spirits were raised by the next patient who presented the symptoms of acute otitis media and had a bulging red tympanic membrane. He was aged three and Dr Preston prescribed amoxycillin, which he knew would be active against *Haemophilus influenzae* which could be a special problem in young children with otitis media, and would also be active against the other common pathogens implicated in this infection. He sat back somewhat relieved that he could apply his scientific knowledge to at least one of the problems presented to him.

His next patient did little to maintain his high spirits. She was a model who had noticed a few spots on her face (Fig. 1.3). With the help of a magnifying glass he was able to confirm her finding but had little to offer to remove the blemish. This was in contrast to the subsequent patient who complained of back pain which was interfering with his work as a labourer but appeared to be unaware of any blemishes on his skin which was peppered with cystic acne (Fig. 1.4).

And so it went on until 11 o'clock by which time he had seen about 20 patients. As he reflected on the morning surgery he tried to analyse the patients he had seen. There were three or four who clearly did not need to consult a

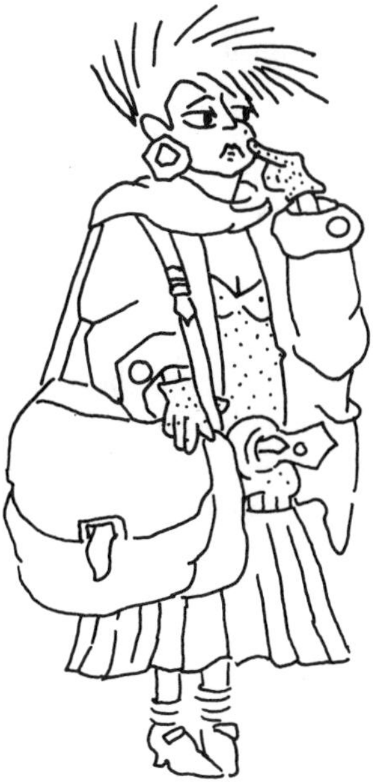

Fig. 1.3.

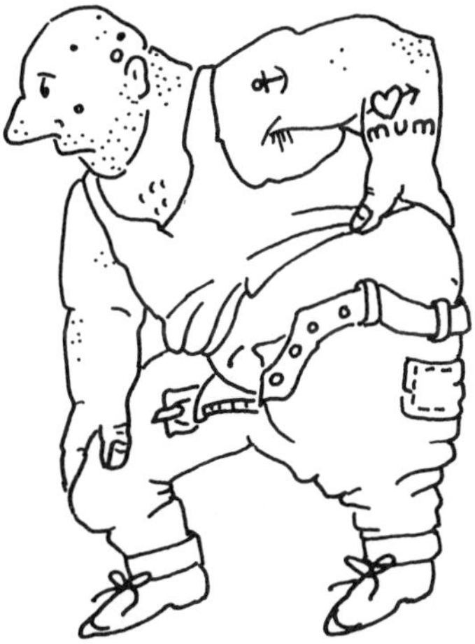

Fig. 1.4.

doctor, but needed to learn how to manage the common symptoms of illness at home. There were some others with similar symptoms which were used to present much more serious problems concerned with their personal relationships. There were yet others presenting illness which could not be explained without reference to their psycho-social background. There were those presenting with serious organic disease and in particular the old lady who had tolerated severe disability because 'the doctor was so busy'. And finally there were the follow-up consultations for chronic disease, some of which reflected organic disease which needed monitoring and some of which reflected the need for the patients to have an illness to explain their behaviour in response to their personal and environmental problems.

In his reverie Dr Preston had forgotten the meeting over coffee to allocate the day's visits. He need not have worried because when he got to the coffee meeting he found that the visits had already been allocated. The senior partner had to go to a trainers' meeting, the second partner had his occupational health work to do, and the third partner was teaching undergraduates, so six of the ten new calls had been allocated to Dr Preston. He was not surprised. It seemed to him as he thought about it rather cynically that the provision of primary care figured fairly low in the priorities of some general practitioners. As he thought about this in his car, he realized that perhaps this was one of the problems of general practice, too much of the decision-making is purely selfish and there is a lack of proper management.

He completed his visits by 1.30p.m. and went home to lunch. Three visits had been calls from old ladies living alone. Each wanted a visit from the doctor. One needed a visit and he admitted her into hospital with pneumonia. One was lonely, isolated, and suffering pain from arthritis. She was very deaf and accepted this as normal at her age. She had received no advice on modern hearing aids and he promised to refer her to the hearing-aid department at the local hospital. The third had fallen over the dog which she had failed to see (Fig. 1.5). Both she and the dog were shocked but otherwise undamaged. He examined her eyes and found that she had advanced cataracts.

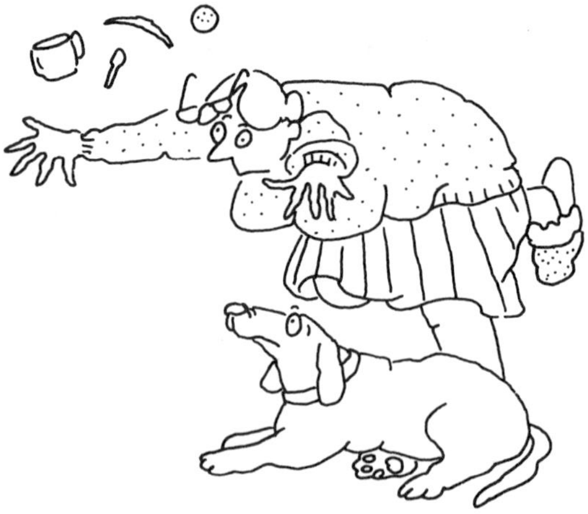

Fig. 1.5.

The other three visits were to children. One had acute otitis media identical to the child he had seen in the surgery. There was a baby who had been vomiting for 12 hours and a five-year-old with a rash. He was left pondering on the difference between medical demand and medical need.

Mrs Preston is a teacher and during lunch they talked about health education and how they could help patients to know more about their health and be better informed about when it is appropriate to consult a doctor. They thought perhaps they should prepare and try out a booklet advising patients about the home treatment of the common minor illnesses, and when a doctor should be called.

After lunch Dr Preston went back to the surgery and wrote up the patients' records and dictated some letters to the secretary. As he was dictating, she intimated to him that he seemed to refer more patients to hospital than the senior partners and wondered why this was. He could think of a variety of explanations, such as that he saw more patients, saw more of the emergencies, or even that as a doctor new from hospital work he identified more quickly the resources available in hospital for high-technology care to relieve the patient's symptoms.

He had an hour to spare before starting the evening surgery and spent some time with the newly appointed practice manager, discussing with her the appointment system, and how it failed to work, and the role of the receptionist in protecting the doctor from unnecessary demands. They even got on to discussing the preventive care provided within the practice and the totally haphazard way of ensuring that patients had regular cervical cytology and the way that comprehensive family planning and well baby care was provided. She saw this as essentially a management problem which could be solved if there was a reliable way of collecting, storing, and retrieving information. She was all into computers.

The evening surgery produced the usual mix of new problems, chronic and totally undiagnosable disease. During the surgery Dr Preston pondered on his discussion with the practice manager and wondered if he should be trying to screen all the patients for such problems as hypertension and breast lumps. He knew that some doctors suggested that this could be built into the routine surgery consultation and this was called 'case-finding' rather than screening. He was not quite clear about the difference but tried out his new case-finding on an obese 50-year-old man who consulted him about a pain in his back. The patient's blood pressure was 170/105. This finding did not help Dr Preston to manage the backache for which he prescribed an analgesic, but it did make him question whether or not he should tell the patient he was hypertensive. Dr Preston remembered vaguely terms like specificity and sensitivity in relation to clinical observations and how they had something to do with false-positive and false-negative findings. He also recalled that most clinical variables are normally distributed about a mean value for the population and hoped that his patient was at the upper limit of the normal distribution. He did not really quite know what this meant but he did not want to confront the patient with raised blood pressure when he had come to him complaining of backache. Dr Preston began to have doubts about the value of case-finding and decided to read up more about it when he returned home.

This problem raised its ugly head later in the surgery. A patient who had presented one week earlier with strange abdominal pains had been submitted to a battery of haemotological and chemical pathology tests. The only abnormal result was a rather low value for the serum potassium. This finding did not in any way contribute to an understanding of the patient's symptoms, so Dr Preston asked her what she thought might be causing her pain. She said she did not know but volunteered the information that her brother had recently been operated on for cancer of the colon and said she was worried that she might be suffering from the same problem. It seemed that the patient's health beliefs and fears might be more valuable in advancing the diagnosis than the blood tests. Dr Preston still did not know quite what to do about the low serum potassium, but somewhere in the distant past he recalled a statistician explaining that if you carried out enough tests, normal variation being what it is, one in twenty would fall outside the normal range. He decided that the patient's potassium level was the one in twenty and reassured her about carcinoma of the colon.

As he drove home that evening he began to question what is meant by normal. It is difficult enough to describe this in the context of blood pressure or serum potassium. It becomes much more difficult when you move into the field of human behaviour. Why did one patient with acute otitis media require a surgery consultation and an identical case demand a home visit? Dr Preston was on call that night and when he was called out at 11.00p.m. to see a child with coryza and at 2.00a.m. to see a child in an acute asthmatic attack which had been in progress for six hours, but for which the parents did not like to bother him, he had still not resolved this problem.

THE EPILOGUE (DR PRESTON'S DAY)

In the course of a single day, Dr Preston identified many of the problems which exercise the minds of new doctors entering general practice. Most of these problems seem insoluble and in the context of the day-to-day pressures on the general practitioner it is often more comfortable to suppress these questions than to face up to them. Those doctors who do face up to them become rapidly aware that they do not have all the resources to answer them. This book is concerned with the knowledge and skills needed to solve some of the problems which Dr Preston identified. What are those problems?

Perhaps the most arresting problem which arose was that of relating patients' demands to patients' needs. Estimates of need may be derived from studies of morbidity in general practice, but they are influenced to such an extent by the local characteristics of the practice that nationally collected data are of limited value. Dr Preston illustrated their limitations further by the difficulty he had in recording the patients' presenting symptoms in terms of their real problems. So the individual general practitioner who wishes to predict his patients' needs must be able to measure certain characteristics of his practice, including the age, sex, and socio-economic status of the patients for whom he is providing care. If he wishes to relate these needs to his patients' demands, he must also be able to measure these demands made upon him. How many of these are initiated by the doctor? Dr Preston wondered why patients with hypertension were seen every two months and not every three or six months. This raises a whole lot of issues about what constitutes optimal care for patients suffering from different diseases. Dr Preston also identified what he felt was inappropriate demand for care. To what extent is this due to doctors inculcating unrealistic expectations in their patients? Can this be modified by patient education?

The appropriateness or otherwise of appointment systems and how they can be controlled was raised by Dr Preston. This problem is complex. It is concerned with the way patients perceive the urgency of their needs for care, the amount of time doctors are prepared to allocate to surgery consultations, and, perhaps above all, the communication between patients and receptionists. Its resolution requires facts about demand for care in relation to the resources provided and about the attitudes of doctors and receptionists in responding to patient demand.

In the diagnostic field, Dr Preston kept coming up against the concept of normality. This included the normal distribution of physical characteristics. Quite separately it raised the issue of normal human behaviour. From the former arises the theory of probability. This includes probability that specific symptoms indicate disease, probability in relation to prognosis, and probability in relation to normal values. The latter concerned with human behaviour is a more complex issue and is related to social, psychological, and cultural norms.

Dr Preston became aware during the day of the pros and cons of screening and case-finding and felt that he should know more about such terms as sensitivity and specificity. He seemed to be impressed that many of the problems in general practice could be solved by better management based on good information, but the question remained as to how good information could be provided and how it could be interpreted.

This is what this book is all about. It is hoped that it will help Dr Preston to answer his problems. He will need to acquire some more knowledge of the epidemiological approach and will have to know how to measure some of the factors which contribute to the problems he perceives and how to interpret the information he collects. He will need to learn about the normal distribution of physical characteristics and human behaviour and how to measure variation from the mean value and what this means. In carrying out experiments in his practice he will need to learn how to turn a question into a testable hypothesis and how to design a study to test this in the hurly-burly of general practice.

It is clear from Dr Preston's day that he also has problems with his partners. This book is not designed to solve the personal relationship problems between partners, but it is hoped that it will provide Dr Preston with the knowledge and skill to accumulate the facts he needs to convince his partners that good management decisions reached in a democratic way will lead to a happy working relationship.

It would be a mistake to conclude from this description of Dr Preston's day that he is unhappy in his work as a general practitioner. He likes Wincampton, he has a happy marriage, and two lovely children. On the whole he gets on well with his partners and the staff in the practice. He gets great emotional satisfaction from the way he has been accepted as a new doctor in the community and from the gratitude of his patients. He does however sometimes feel that his medical education did not prepare him adequately to deal with the problems he encounters. He suspects that a better understanding of epidemiology would help him to deal with problems which are inevitable in a system of primary care which is freely accessible to the population.

2 What is happening to me?

David Morrell

Dr Preston feels trapped by the demands which are being made on him. He can remain trapped throughout his professional life, or he can try to stand back and review objectively the situation. To do this he must escape from his anecdotal descriptions of his workload and develop methods of measuring it.

The first measure he will wish to make is that of his consultation rate. He will want at first to compare this with consultation rates recorded by other general practitioners locally and nationally, and in due course may wish to compare his consultation rate with that of his partners.

CONSULTATION RATE

The consultation rate measures the number of consultations which take place in relation to the population which is generating these consultations, and which will be referred to in future as the population at risk. It may be expressed as follows:

$$\text{Consultation rate} = \frac{\text{consultations per year}}{\text{practice population}}$$

This measures the number of consultations per year per patient registered with the practice. The national rate is in the region of 3.5 consultations per patient per year. A number of problems arise however in calculating the consultation rates.

The denominator

The denominator of the formula is the population to which the doctors are at risk. This may be described by the population registered with the practice at the Family Practitioner Committee (FPC). The size of the population is returned at three monthly intervals by the FPC and the number of patients over 65 and 75 years old is also recorded.

These returns, however, provide no information about the age or sex distribution of the patients in the practice under the age of 65 years. A few FPCs will provide a full age and sex breakdown of registered patients. In the near future it is hoped that all FPCs will provide this facility. Most practitioners who wish to determine the age and sex distribution of the patients registered with them are at present constrained to create their own age/sex register.

Though it is time-consuming to create an age/sex register, it is a necessary preliminary to looking critically at a practice. It is for instance impossible to compare the consultation rates of an individual practice with national data unless the age and sex of the patients in the practice can be compared with the population from which the national data are derived.

Creating an age/sex register

Creating an age/sex register means extracting information about the surname, forename, sex, and date of birth from all the medical records of the patients held in the practice. To this basic information should be added the name of the doctor with whom the patient is registered, because this information makes it possible to compare the practice register with the FPC register which is filed by the doctor. If the practice records are exceptionally well kept, the marital status and occupation of the patient may be added, but this information is rarely readily available and needs constant updating. These data are then transferred either to a ledger in which each page represents a year of birth, or to a card index which is filed by year of birth, or to a computer. Suitable cards (blue for males, pink for females) are produced by the Royal College of General Practitioners (RCGP). Once the register is compiled it can be used to relate consultations to the practice population in terms of specified age groups and by sex.

There are however some problems with age/sex registers compiled in this way. When new patients join the practice, their names will immediately be added to the register. When patients leave the practice, however, their names will only be deleted when their records are recalled by the FPC. The practice register will therefore always be inflated by the numbers of patients who have left the practice, but who have not re-registered with another general practitioner. This inflation, however, is to some extent balanced by the number of individuals living in the community to whom the practice is at risk, but who will not register for care until they fall ill. In practices where the age and sex of patients immigrating and emigrating is similar, this is not a serious problem, but where these two groups differ it may produce important anomalies. In addition, in nearly all practice filing systems there are notes of patients who have gone abroad, or who on re-registering with a doctor have not been able to recall the name of their previous general practitioner, and even some who have died or entered old people's homes in another area and have not been notified to the practice. These dead files represent 5–10 per cent of most practice files and these figures may be even higher where the population is very mobile.

Consultation rates in partnerships

A single-handed doctor can count the number of consultations he undertakes and divide this by the population registered with him to give an annual consultation rate and he can subdivide this to give rates for specific age and sex groups. In only a minority of partnerships do doctors consult only with their own registered patients. In most, patients are given freedom to consult with the partner of their choice, and over a period of years the patients consulting a particular doctor may not represent the patients registered with that doctor. In this situation it is very difficult to calculate the consultation rates of a particular doctor because no denominator is available. This is the situation which appears to exist in Dr Preston's practice. He will be able to calculate the consultation rates of the partners in relation to the overall practice population, but will not be able to relate this directly to the population for which the individual doctors are responsible.

In countries where patients do not have to register for primary care it is not possible to construct an age/sex register. In this situation the alternative is to count the total number of patients consulting in the year analysed by age and sex. The consultation rate per patient consulting may then be calculated from the following formula:

$$\text{Consultation rate per patient consulting} = \frac{\text{total consultations}}{\text{number of patients consulting}}$$

This may be useful in comparing consultation rates over two periods of time to determine changes in workload, or patient or doctor behaviour, but is of less value than the consultation rate per registered patient, because it ignores those who do not consult at all, which in some age groups may be up to 40 per cent of the population.

What is a consultation?

Determining the denominator presents some problems in calculating consultation rates. Measuring the numerator, the number of consultations is not entirely straightforward either. It is important in studying demand in general practice to define clearly what is meant by a consultation. Most commonly it is considered to imply a meeting face-to-face between patient and doctor. This excludes telephone consultations which can account for an important part of the doctor's work and are likely to vary widely between doctors. Where do repeat prescriptions ordered at reception and completed by the doctor fit into this record of demand? Should home visits and out-of-hours consultations be considered separately? The Research Unit at Birmingham of the RCGP (1973) has drawn up a scheme of definitions to deal with these problems, and it is important for Dr Preston to abide by these if he hopes to compare his findings with the work of other general practitioners.

The importance of differentiating between patient- and doctor-initiated consultations was pointed out by Morrell (1971). The patient-initiated consultation is one in which the patient makes the decision to consult and is thus a true reflection of demand for general practitioner care. These normally account for about 50 per cent of the workload and are not directly under the control of the doctor. The doctor-initiated consultation occurs because the doctor has told the patient to consult again after a period of time or to consult again if no better. The doctor may also constrain the patient to consult again by prescribing drugs for a limited period of time or by issuing a certificate for a specified time period. Doctors may markedly increase their workload by asking patients to return at frequent intervals and Dr Preston wondered about this in the management of patients with hypertension. This may reflect a doctor's concern for his patients or a doctor's insecurity. Sometimes it reflects the fact that the doctor has not thought clearly about what he wishes to achieve at the return consultation. This is clearly something which Dr Preston should examine if he wishes to compare the behaviour of the doctors within a partnership. It is not unheard of for young doctors to accuse their senior partners of bringing back patients with chronic and undemanding problems for return consultations in order to protect themselves from new and more demanding problems. Hopefully Dr Preston will not make such claims without good evidence.

Another type of doctor-initiated consultation is that concerned with prevention. Regular antenatal and well baby clinics fit into this definition, as also do many consultations for contraception, cervical cytology, and screening for some other disorders. In studying general practice it may be desirable to analyse these consultations separately.

How to study demand for general practitioner care

Once consultation rates have been measured, the doctor may become curious about the content and outcome of the consultation and wish to record this. The method used for studying consultations will depend to some extent on the way the practice is organized. The single-handed doctor may simply keep a diary of all his consultations, and this can subsequently be analysed. In partnership practices where several doctors are collecting information, it is important to agree the definitions which will be used. If the practice is using an appointment system, the simplest method of recording data is for the receptionists, at the start of each surgery, to prepare an encounter sheet for each doctor. This lists the names, dates of birth, and sex of the patients booked for the consulting session. Blank columns may then be left for the doctor to record other information about the consultation, depending on the object of the study. A space to indicate whether the consultation is initiated by the patient or doctor according to an agreed definition is very useful. Spaces may also be provided for the doctor to record the problem presented and the diagnosis and possibly to include information about hospital referrals, prescribing, etc. (see Fig. 2.1).

Patients attending the session without an appointment may be added to the list, possibly in red ink so that they can be counted separately, and patients who fail to keep their appointments identified in some agreed way. The encounter sheets may subsequently be analysed by a receptionist or secretary in terms of the age and sex of the patients consulting, the number of unbooked attenders and defaulters, and whatever other variables the doctors consider important. These data can be analysed manually or, if a computer is available,

DATE DOCTOR

NAME	Sex	Date of Birth	Type Of Consultation	DIAGNOSIS 1	DIAGNOSIS 2	DIAGNOSIS 3	REFERRAL Investigation	REFERRAL Specialist	REFERRAL Nurse	REFERRAL Social Worker	EXAMINATION None	ENT	Chest	CVS	Abdomen	Joints	CNS	Skin	Eye	PR	PV

Fig. 2.1. Encounter sheet.

fed daily into the computer and subsequently analysed. Information about home visits must also be recorded, most conveniently in a ledger which the doctors complete following the visit, and the same system may be applied for out-of-hours care. Repeat prescriptions are normally requested through the receptionist and these data may most conveniently be recorded by the receptionists.

Missing data

The amount and complexity of the data collected in general practice is almost invariably inversely related to the accuracy and completeness of the data collected. Consultations in general practice occur at intervals of six to seven minutes and, during this time, the doctor has to make a variety of decisions. If he is also constrained to complete complex records for research purposes, he will almost certainly fail to do so when he is under pressure. For this reason, when Dr Preston is studying demand in his practice, he would be well advised to keep the recording as simple as possible and to put the onus on ensuring complete recording on his clerical staff. On the whole, they are much better at co-operating in such activities than doctors and they can be trained to monitor the recording of the doctors. Very many studies of general practice have produced worthless results because the data collected have been incomplete. A well-trained secretary or receptionist, or in major studies a research assistant, can monitor on a day-to-day basis the data collected, can gently or not so gently prompt doctors who are failing to play their part, and if they monitor the records within 24 hours of the consultation can sometimes retrieve missing data. If complete and accurate information is required, such an assistant is well worth the investment.

MORBIDITY RECORDING

Doctors who study the demands made on them may, in due course, wish to study, in more detail, the illnesses presented to them. This may be because they are interested in following the natural history of some particular illness, or because they are interested in the overall pattern of morbidity in general practice. Some studies may be motivated primarily to improve the care provided for particular diseases or to organize it more efficiently. Others may be concerned with advancing knowledge about the incidence, natural history, or outcome of disease. In any of these situations the doctor must face the problems of recording morbidity in general practice.

It is likely that in due course Dr Preston will wish to record the sort of problems presented in his practice and possibly to relate these to his patients' needs. This introduces him to recording morbidity data in general practice.

Patients initiate consultations with general practitioners for a wide variety of reasons. These patient-initiated consultations represent new problems about which the patient wishes to consult. These problems are normally presented as symptoms of illness. The relationship between the symptoms presented and the problem identified is often obscure, and the concept that an accurate history of the symptoms, complemented by the appropriate physical examination, with or without investigation, will lead to a diagnosis is an illusion derived from the rather simplistic diagnostic process taught to undergraduates. The two situations in which patients present their problems, primary care (general practice) and secondary care (hospital practice), are very different. In the former it is determined by a lay decision, that of the patient, who is anxious about changes he has noticed in his bodily structure or function. These changes have usually been present for a short period of time, i.e. hours or days. The patient attending hospital is usually there because the doctor is anxious, i.e. a professional judgement has been made which qualifies the patient for a second opinion. With the exception of emergencies, the symptoms have usually been present for a much longer period of time, have been assessed as probably representing a serious pathological process, and the probability that a definitive clinical diagnosis will be reached is very much higher.

In contrast, doctor-initiated consultations in general practice are usually concerned either with the continuing care of chronic disease or with follow-up consultations demanded by some acute illnesses. A clear diagnosis is much more likely to be forthcoming in these situations. Unfortunately many patients suffering from chronic disease suffer from more than one disease and a decision as to the particular problem leading to the consultation may be obscure.

For these reasons morbidity recording in general practice is never straightforward. National morbidity studies conducted in general practice, e.g. RCGP, OPCS, DHSS (1986), describe the consultation rates for different age and sex groups in the population, and the diagnoses recorded at these consultations are based on information collected by a selected group of general practitioners who are willing to record data at every consultation over a long period of time. It is clearly not possible in a large morbidity survey to define every diagnosis recorded. It therefore follows that the diagnoses recorded by individual doctors reflect their subjective response to the symptoms and signs presented. There is inevitably, as Dr Preston observed, a pressure on the doctors involved to reach a diagnosis and, as he rightly pointed out, at many consultations in general practice this is not possible. For this reason some studies of morbidity in general practice have focused on symptoms presented at a new consultation or on the problems which the general practitioner identifies rather than on a conventional medical diagnosis. This is discussed in more detail in Chapter 7.

Once data have been collected, it is necessary to code them in some way so that they can be analysed. In many of the early studies of morbidity in general practice attempts were made to apply the International Classification of Diseases (ICD) index (WHO 1975) to morbidity data collected in general practice. This was found to be difficult. The reason for this was that the ICD index was developed for hospital and death certification data and could not readily be applied to the diagnoses which often did not proceed beyond the symptomatic level in general practice. As a result the RCGP Research Unit in Birmingham developed a much simplified coding system which has been widely used and regularly updated (RCGP 1984). The World Organization of National Colleges and Academies of General Practice (WONCAGP) tried to improve on this and to produce a coding system acceptable on an international basis known as the International Classification of Health Problems in Primary Care (WONCAGP 1979). Primary care varies so widely throughout the world that it is questionable whether an internationally acceptable coding system will ever be achieved and the RCGP's classification is probably still the most useful for practitioners working in the UK. With the introduction of computers to primary care a variety of other coding systems are being introduced which complicates an already confused situation.

The doctor who wishes to measure the pattern of illness presented in his practice by some form of morbidity recording should think very carefully about the questions he wishes to answer before plunging into a detailed morbidity study of his consultation data. He may find it helpful in clarifying his objectives to answer the following questions:

1. What are the important problems and how will the data collected help to solve these problems?
2. Will the data collected be sufficiently complete and sufficiently well defined and accurate to be interpreted?
3. What is the easiest way of collecting the data needed to answer the problems in my practice?
4. How will the data be collected, coded, and analysed, and what are the implications of this in terms of practice workload?
5. How likely is it that the data collected will lead to changes in the methods of providing care?

To answer these questions the doctor may need help from an epidemiologist or statistician. Having answered these questions he will be in a better position to decide on the type of study he wishes to carry out in his practice. Two methods of morbidity recording are described:

(1) full morbidity recording;
(2) selective recording of morbidity.

Full morbidity recording

This demands that at each consultation occurring in the practice a diagnosis or problem is recorded. These diagnoses are subsequently analysed in a way which is designed to answer the practitioner's particular questions.

A number of methods have been devised for collecting this type of information. Using the standard National Health Service (NHS) form, FP8, the doctor may box in his diagnosis at each consultation (Fig. 2.2). A receptionist or secretary may then subsequently review the records at the end of the consulting session and extract this information. In some practices using A4 records, a separate column is reserved for the diagnosis of the patient's main problem. In the example illustrated (Fig. 2.3), this problem column is placed on a continuation sheet which is immediately exposed when the record is opened, thus facilitating the extraction of information (Fig. 2.4). In most morbidity studies, however, a special encounter sheet is developed on which the data is recorded.

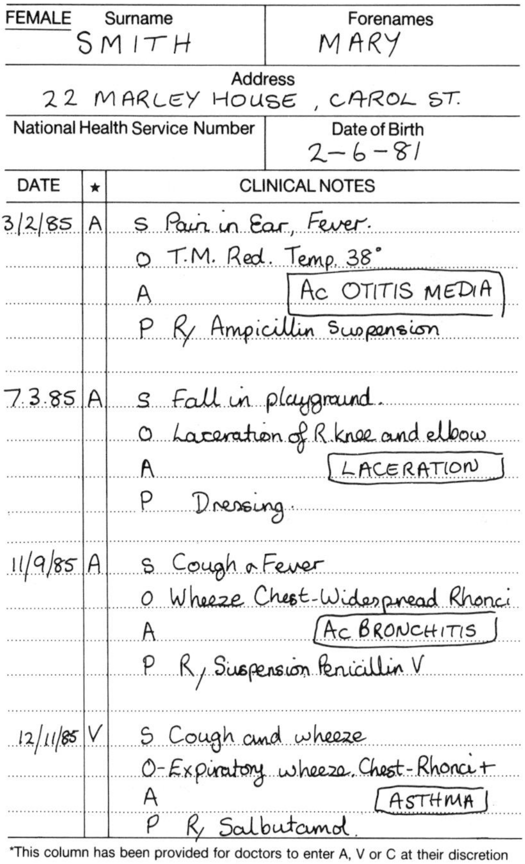

FEMALE Surname SMITH | Forenames MARY

Address 22 MARLEY HOUSE, CAROL ST.

National Health Service Number | Date of Birth 2-6-81

DATE	★	CLINICAL NOTES
3/2/85	A	S Pain in Ear, Fever.
		O T.M. Red. Temp. 38°
		A [Ac OTITIS MEDIA]
		P Rx Ampicillin Suspension
7.3.85	A	S Fall in playground.
		O Laceration of R knee and elbow
		A [LACERATION]
		P Dressing.
11/9/85	A	S Cough & Fever
		O Wheeze Chest-Widespread Rhonci
		A [Ac BRONCHITIS]
		P Rx Suspension Penicillin V
12/11/85	V	S Cough and wheeze
		O-Expiratory wheeze. Chest-Rhonci +
		A [ASTHMA]
		P Rx Salbutamol.

*This column has been provided for doctors to enter A, V or C at their discretion

Fig. 2.2. Form E.C.8 Diagnosis boxed in for subsequent extraction.

The way the data are extracted will be determined to a large extent by the purpose of the study. If the doctor is simply interested in describing the pattern of illness encountered in his practice, e.g. to understand how often particular problems present, the diagnosis will simply be related to the overall number of consultations. In many cases, however, e.g. in planning care, he will be

12837

Date	S/V/O	½	CONSULTATION DATA	PROBLEM	No.
			OCCUPATION Taxi Driver		
			MARITAL STATUS Married		
2/4/86	S	2	S – Sympton free	DIABETES	1
			O Home test. Blood sugars 7–11	MELLITUS	
			BP 170/100. Fundi ✓ Pulses ✓ Urine ✓	Hypertension	2
			P. ℞ Atanolol 100mg Daily		
			Insulatard 20U. AM		
			16U. PM		
3/7/86	S	1	S – Rash on hands Decorating bedroom	Contact	3
			O – Eczematous rash on hands and wrists	Eczema	
			P – Advice		
			℞ 1% Hydrocortisone Cream		
4/10/86	S	2	P. ℞ Influvac	Immunisation	1
8/12/86	S	1	S – Cough, fever, yellow spit, breathless		
			O – T37	Ac BRONCHITIS	4
			Chest – Prolonged Expiration. Widespread râles e rhonci		
			BP 160/100 Blood sugars 10–14		
			P ℞ Amoxycillin 250mg + ds. cc.		

Fig. 2.3. Consultation sheet from A4 records illustrating a 'problem' column.

interested in relating the diagnosis recorded to the characteristics of the patients presenting, such as age and sex, and possibly to the type of consultation, i.e. doctor- or patient-initiated. Almost invariably, he will wish to analyse the diagnostic information into broad categories and for this it is necessary to code the data recorded. A typical extraction sheet for this type of study is illustrated in Fig. 2.5.

In many studies of morbidity, the doctor is interested in linking the diagnosis to the individual patient with a view to subsequently identifying particular groups for more detailed study or identifying particularly vulnerable groups for preventive care. It was for this purpose that the 'E book' was developed, named after its inventor, Dr T. Eimeryl. This provides a loose-leaf ledger with a page for each of 500 diagnostic codings derived from the RCGP's (1975) *Classification of diseases, infections and causes of death.* The names and NHS numbers of patients suffering from these diseases are entered on a separate interleafed sheet and thus lists of patients who have been diagnosed as suffering from particular diseases can easily be extracted.

The computer is now rapidly replacing the E book and most practices interested in morbidity studies either possess their own microcomputer or have access to one. If a practice owns a computer, data may be typed directly

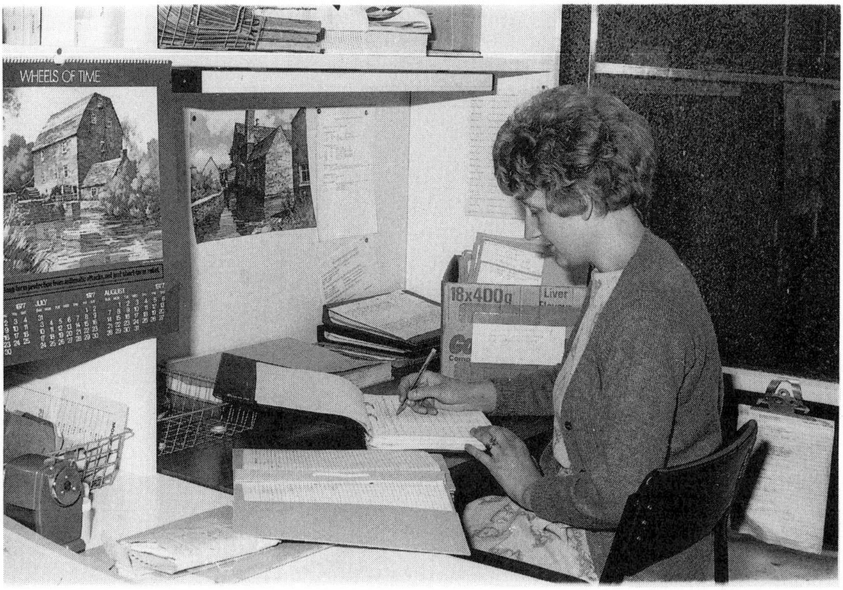

Fig. 2.4.

from the medical record or encounter sheet into the computer. Alternatively, extracted data may be sent in batches to a central computer for recording and analysis.

Limited morbidity recording

In situations where the doctor is concerned primarily with identifying groups suffering from particular disorders, such as diabetes or hypertension, for either research purposes or in order to provide continuing care, he may decide to limit his morbidity recording to specific diagnoses. In its most simple form this has been achieved very effectively by attaching coloured stickers to the records of patients suffering from particular disorders, a system initiated by the RCGP some 25 years ago.

This method, however, is very limited and it is apparent that there are many chronic illnesses or important operations or allergies which should be clearly identified on a patient's records and could usefully be recorded on a practice register. Zander *et al.* (1978) introduced the concept of a chronic problem list. These problems were defined as 'Problems of a permanent nature which influence the care of the patients for the rest of their lives'. They developed a list of problems which were encompassed by this definition and to which a secretary or receptionist may refer when extracting data from ongoing records. The groups of problems are summarized below:

1. Conditions relevant to the assessment of a patient's current problem:
   (a) conditions liable to remission or recurrence,

Patient number:

Date:

Date of birth:

Sex (male 1, female 2):

Type of Consultation (Doctor-initiated 1) (Patient-initiated 2)

Diagnosis 1
2
3

Referral-Investigation
Specialist
Nurse
Social worker

Examination-None
ENT
Chest
CVS
Abdomen
Joints
CNS
Skin
Eye
PR
PV

Fig. 2.5.

e.g. peptic ulcer, disseminated sclerosis;

(b) conditions liable to complications,
e.g. malignancy/potential malignancy, alcoholism;

(c) major operations;

(d) important conditions which the patient might be reluctant to make known, e.g. venereal disease, attempted suicide.

2. Conditions requiring continuing medical care:

(a) conditions needing long-term management,
e.g. hypertension, pernicious anaemia;

(b) conditions needing long-term follow-up,
e.g. renal insufficiency, partial gastrectomy, thyrotoxicosis treated with I^{131}.

3. Conditions affecting choice of drug: e.g. allergies and sensitivities, peptic ulcer, (aspirin), valvular heart disease (antibiotics).
4. Conditions affecting patient's function, e.g. blindness, phobic anxiety state, senile dementia.

A typical summary problem list retained in the patient's record and on the computer register is illustrated in Fig. 2.6.

SUMMARY PROBLEM LIST

	Date		PROBLEM	ACTION
	1979	1	THYROTOXICOSIS, I^{131}	Annual Thyroid Function
	1981	2	HYSTERECTOMY (Fibroids)	
	1983	3	HYPERTENSION	See flowchart
	1985	4	PENICILLIN ALLERGY	
	1986	5	PERNICIOUS ANAEMIA	Annual Blood Count

Fig. 2.6. Summary problem list.

Comparative studies

In due course, Dr Preston may wish to compare the results of his studies with national and regional data. In doing so he will need to answer some important questions:

1. How does the population in my practice compare in terms of age, sex, and possibly social class with a population studied in a national morbidity study?
2. How does my practice in terms of environmental factors, such as urban vs. rural setting, differ from the practices in the national survey?
3. What were the methods of data collection in the national survey?
4. What definitions were used in collecting the data?
5. What precautions were taken to avoid missing data or recording inaccurate data?

6. How were the data coded?

Clearly it is very much better to ask these questions before carrying out a morbidity study in general practice because the answers may influence the design of the study. It may be possible to design a study which is closely comparable in terms of items 3–6. The population characteristics may differ, however, and before comparisons can be made it is necessary to manipulate the data in such a way that the population differences can be minimized.

This means that the data collected in the practice must be expressed in terms of different age, sex, and if possible social class groups and compared with the national data expressed in the same way. This is illustrated in Table 2.1.

Table 2.1.

Age groups	Consultation rates per year			
	Practice study		National study	
	Males	Females	Males	Females
0–4	5.6	5.2	4.8	4.4
5–14	3.8	3.6	3.2	3.0
15–24	2.8	5.8	2.0	4.3

An individual practice is a microcosm of the sort of population used for national studies and is likely to differ in a variety of local, environmental, and population characteristics from the national study. Observed differences must therefore be treated with great care. They may indeed reflect a difference in workload, but interpreting this in terms of the population or practice characteristics is hazardous.

REFERENCES

Morrell, D. C. (1971). Expressions of morbidity in general practice. *British Medical Journal* **2,** 454.

RCGP (Royal College of General Practitioners) (1973). A general practice glossary. *Journal of the Royal College of General Practitioners* **23,** suppl. 3.

RCGP (Royal College of General Practitioners) (1984). Classification of diseases, problems and procedures. *Journal of the Royal College of General Practitioners.* Occasional Paper 26.

RCGP, OPCS, DHSS (Royal College of General Practitioners, Office of Population Censuses and Surveys, Department of Health and Social Security) (1986). Morbidity statistics from general practice 1981–82. *HMSO Series MB5, no. 1.*

WHO (World Health Organization) (1978). *Manual of the international statistical classification of diseases, infections and causes of death. Ninth review.* WHO, Geneva.

WONCAGP (World Organization of National Colleges and Academies of General

Practice) (1979). *An international classification of the health problems of primary care* (ICHPPC-2). Oxford University Press.

Zander, L., Beresford, S., and Thomas, P. (1978). *Medical records in general practice. Journal of the Royal College of General Practitioners*, Occasional Paper 5, pp. 6–15.

3 What are my patients' needs?

David Morrell

Dr Preston, like many of his colleagues, repeatedly questioned whether the demands made on him as a general practitioner really reflected the needs of his practice population. The fact that one patient presented in his surgery with symptoms identical to those which led another to request a home visit perplexed him. He was distressed that some elderly patients tolerated as normal major disabilities produced by defects in vision and hearing, and even apologized for presenting the classical symptoms of cardiac failure. He was surprised how physical symptoms of illness could reflect such serious social and interpersonal relationship problems which were quite unamenable to care by the application of normal medical procedures. Many of the factors which influence the translation of perceived symptoms to demands for medical care are considered in Chapter 7. This chapter focuses on the problems of measuring need for care.

MEASURING MEDICAL NEED

Epidemiologists are often considered unnecessarily pedantic in demanding that words, statements, and questions should be clearly defined. It is important to bear in mind that epidemiology is concerned with measurement and with attempting to quantify such things as the incidence or prevalence of disease or disability in populations. General practitioners, such as Dr Preston, who have the same end in view, i.e. quantifying the medical needs of a defined population of patients, must accept the same discipline. In tackling this problem, it is necessary to be clear what is meant by such words as health, disease, illness, and sickness, because these words are all used in different ways in describing the needs of individuals for health care.

Health

Definitions of health have been singularly unsuccessful. The World Health Organization's definition of 'complete physical, mental and social well-being and not merely the absence of disease and infirmity' (WHO Constitution, 1948) excludes most individuals from describing themselves as healthy. From the point of view of therapeutic goals, health is more conveniently thought of as the optimum adaptation of the individual to his environments, physical, psychological, and social. Within this definition the individual's health depends not only on his personal resources in adapting to disability, but on the environment in which he lives. Manipulation of this environment is mainly a responsibility of society, although the doctor may intervene at times to influence the role of society or to change the immediate environment of the individual. He is however always concerned in supporting the individual in his physical and psychological response to disability and can sometimes modify the physical aspects of the problem.

Disease

This describes a pathological process most often associated with physical changes. It may be quite clear-cut as in the physical changes brought about by trauma, infection, or malignancy. In some cases, however, it is much less clearly defined. If disease is a deviation from structural and functional biological normality, it raises the whole question of what is normal. Many physical characteristics such as blood pressure, body weight, and blood sugar are continuously distributed and there is no clear point at which health turns into disease. Disease in these cases is negotiated in relation to such factors as the prognostic significance of the measurement at a particular point in time in the life span of the individual. This is discussed in more detail in Chapter 4.

Illness

This is a feeling, an experience which is personal to the patient. It may be accompanied by disease and in these cases reflects the effects of the disease on the individual's feelings and function. Sometimes illness is experienced where there is no evidence of physical disease. This situation presents major problems for doctors trained to relate illness to demonstrable pathology. Illness, however, can cause disability in the absence of disease and can lead to demands for medical care.

Sickness

This is the public or external display of illness or disease. Sickness is a social role or status. It is a recognition by society that the patient is sick and needs to be sustained. At every consultation the doctor is challenged to establish, maintain, or terminate the sick role of his patient. The security of the sick role depends on a number of factors of which an important one is to be in the possession of a disease.

In measuring medical need in general practice it is important to recognize the different ways in which medical need may be expressed, as disability, disease, illness, or sickness. These needs may be expressed overtly in the consultation, but some of them may be tolerated by individuals and never presented to the doctor. Some may be accompanied by disability which could be ameliorated by medical intervention. Others may produce no symptoms but be potential causes of serious illness and disability. With all these problems in mind it may be helpful to try to classify the needs of a population of patients in general practice. In this context symptoms may be defined as deviations from normal health which are perceived by individuals but which may or may not be presented to the doctor.

Acute illness

1. Acute symptomatic disease needing medical care.
Examples include infections such as pneumonia, vascular accidents such as stroke or myocardial infarction, malignant disease, and trauma.

2. Acute symptomatic disease not needing medical care.
Examples include acute diseases such as viral respiratory infections, strains and sprains of the musculo–skeletal system. For these medicine can offer no cure and they may more appropriately be treated by self-care. The need in these cases may be more concerned with reassuring the patient that he is suffering from a common cold and not pneumonia, glandular fever, malaria, or a broken bone. It is in this group of minor illness that cultural and social factors play a major part in determining whether or not illness will lead to a request for care.

3. Acute symptomatic illness not explained by disease.
Such illness may reflect maladaption of the individual to social, environmental, and psychological stress, or the early stages of diseases which are not yet identifiable by normal investigative processes. Many mental illnesses come into this category.

4. Acute symptoms not perceived as illness.
These patients experience deviations from normal health but do not see these as needing medical care. Such symptoms as loss of appetite, weight loss, depression, or constipation may be ignored for many months before a patient seeks care.

Progressive incurable disease

1. Patients experience chronic diseases which need continuing care in general practice. Some of these are seen at regular intervals by the general practitioner, and other patients are told to consult under certain circumstances. Examples include chronic bronchitis, hypertension, osteoarthritis, and schizophrenia.

2. Some patients, particularly those in the older age groups, experience symptoms which they attribute to the ageing process, but which in fact reflect disease processes which are amenable to medical care. These include illnesses presenting such symptoms as deteriorating vision or hearing, increasing shortness of breath, ankle oedema, or weight loss.

Pre-symptomatic disease

Individuals may suffer from pre-symptomatic disease, the prognosis of which can be influenced by medical care. There are two broad groups:

(a) adults with such diseases as asymptomatic hypertension, diabetes, cervical cancer, or glaucoma;
(b) infants and children with developmental abnormality such as hearing and speech delays, squint, congenital heart disease, or congenital dislocation of the hip.

Vulnerable patients

Some individuals are in need of medical supervision because their psychosocial or physical needs make them particularly vulnerable to illness and disease. Examples include patients who have in the past been treated for instance by gastric surgery or radioactive isotopes and need regular monitoring. There are also groups of socially deprived patients such as single parents, the elderly living alone, and those with psychiatric disorders who are particularly vulnerable to illness, sickness, and disability.

METHODS OF MEASURING NEED IN GENERAL PRACTICE POPULATIONS

The foregoing paragraphs summarize the ways in which need for medical care may be defined. Any attempt to measure need in general practice must start with some definition of the need which is to be measured and some estimate of the size of the problem. In this context the terms prevalence and incidence are frequently used by epidemiologists.

Definitions of incidence and prevalence

Incidence

This refers to new events, e.g. new cases of disease and new symptoms occurring in a defined population within a specified period of time.

Prevalence

This refers to the number of cases of a disease or condition which exist in a defined population in a designated period of time; e.g. point prevalence refers to the number of persons with a particular disease at a given point in time, annual prevalence refers to the number of persons known to have a particular disease at any time during a particular year.

The prevalence of symptoms of illness

At its simplest this may refer to symptoms of illness which have been experienced over a finite period of time and this may be related to the action taken by the patients in seeking medical care. An example of this type of study is that by Dunnell and Cartwright (1972) which related symptoms experienced over a two-week period to the drugs consumed and the consultations with doctors. The information was derived from interviews with a random sample of patients to whom a 'questionnaire' was administered. A rather different approach was used by Banks *et al.* (1975) who asked a sample of patients to record in a 'diary' over a period of one month the symptoms they experienced and the action they took in response to these symptoms. Both methods provide some measure of the prevalence of symptoms in the community and the action taken in response to these symptoms. Whether this action was appropriate or not is, to a large extent, a subjective judgement of the researchers.

The prevalence of disease

This demands a very clear definition of what constitutes a 'case' of the particular disease. Some diseases may be defined in terms of the answer to a questionnaire, such as the Medical Research Council questionnaire on chronic bronchitis (MRC 1976) or the general health questionnaire designed to identify 'cases' of psychiatric disorder (Goldberg 1972). In many cases, however, in order to measure the prevalence of a particular disease it is necessary to carry out an objective measurement of physical characteristics such as the level of blood pressure, presence of glycosuria, breast palpation or mammography, respiratory function tests, or electrocardiographs. Most questionnaires are a proxy for clinical examination and have been carefully validated against clinical studies on the basis of which cut-off points are determined to indicate normal or abnormal.

Many of the physical characteristics measured in prevalence studies are continuously distributed in the population and it is necessary to determine in advance the values which differentiate normal from abnormal. In many cases it is also important to determine the conditions under which the tests will be conducted. Will, for instance, the blood pressure be judged as normal or abnormal on the basis of a single reading, or the mean of three readings? Will the pressure be measured after a period of rest and at what intervals of time will the sequence of measurements be carried out?

It is important to differentiate the needs of the epidemiologist in measuring the prevalence of disease or disability from the needs of the general practitioner. The epidemiologist is usually interested in identifying cases in order to relate the disease to the characteristics of the patients and their environment and so to further the knowledge of the aetiology of the disease. His methods must be rigorous, or incorrect conclusions may be reached. The general practitioner may be concerned with identifying patients with a particular disease because he believes that the patient may benefit from treatment. In organizing his practice, adherence to rigid definitions may seem to be relatively unimportant. They are however important if he wishes to generalize from his findings to communicate his conclusions to his colleagues or develop a practice policy for management.

Prevalence of disability

Measurements of disability may be either subjective or objective. The former depend upon a subject's answers to a questionnaire and are usually related to the ability to carry out the normal activities of life. Examples are the Sickness Impact Profile (Bergner and Gibson 1980) and the Nottingham Health Profile (Hunt *et al.* 1985). These subjective measures have been carefully validated by objective findings. Alternatively, disability may be measured directly by observing individuals' ability to perform a variety of tasks, such as climb stairs, read a newspaper, hear the spoken voice at a defined distance, get out of bed or a chair, wash and dress themselves, etc.

Why measure need?

The practitioner may wish to measure the needs of his population for two main reasons:

(1) to quantify these needs prior to deciding how the practice can most appropriately respond to the needs;
(2) to identify all individual patients suffering from a particular need in order to provide a service for them.

These two purposes demand different strategies. In the first, the doctor needs to study a sample of the population which will reflect the needs of the whole population. In the second, he is seeking to identify all the patients in his population with a particular need and is thus constrained to study the entire population. It is sensible to start by studying a sample of the population so that the magnitude of the problem can be measured and on the basis of this an estimate made of the resources needed to study the entire population. In some cases previous studies in general practice can be used to make these estimates, but individual practices may vary widely in their characteristics and it is not always helpful to extrapolate from data collected in one practice in order to predict the situation in another.

STUDYING A SAMPLE OF PATIENTS IN GENERAL PRACTICE

Sampling properly carried out can provide unbiased results and is therefore important in estimating the size of a particular problem in general practice. It has certain real advantages over attempts to survey an entire practice population:

(1) the workload involved in studying a sample is reduced as compared with studying the entire population;
(2) the smaller number of patients to be interviewed or examined reduces the time needed to carry out a study and allows more time to interview or examine each individual;

(3) studying a smaller number of patients makes it possible to ensure that the data are accurately collected and in some cases make it possible to collect more data on each subject.

A study of a sample of the population rather than of the whole population, however, does carry with it one disadvantage, and this is that it introduces a sampling error. This is why it is important to design the study carefully and with the advice of a statistician. If a true random sample of the population is identified for study, the sampling error will not be completely eradicated, but it can be quantified so that the doctor can present his results knowing that the true value for the population will lie within clearly defined limits of confidence.

Random sampling

The great advantage of random sampling is that the results obtained are amenable to statistical interpretation based on the laws of chance. The essential characteristic of random sampling is that everyone in the practice population has an independent and equal chance of appearing in the sample. In sampling from a population such as the general practitioner's list, the easiest way to achieve this is to allot numbers serially to all the patients in the practice. This can be very easily achieved if the practice has an age/sex register on a computer. A table of random sample numbers is then consulted and the point in the table from which the random numbers should be used is determined by chance (such as by marking the table with a pencil with the eyes shut). The series of numbers in the column thus selected is then used to identify the serial numbers of the patients to be studied (detailed instructions on the use of random numbers are provided in the books of random numbers). This method of sampling does not, of itself, ensure that the sample selected is a good sample in the sense that it is representative of the whole population. The play of chance will sometimes produce some unrepresentative samples. Whether or not this occurs is dependent on the sample size. If the sample is large (say 200–300) it is unlikely to be distorted, but if it is small (say 20 or less) it could easily give a very inaccurate estimate. The solution to this problem is therefore to use as big a sample as feasible.

The stratified sample

The population to be sampled may be divided into separate strata, e.g. according to age and sex. A random sample may then be drawn from each stratum and this will ensure that the pre-selected proportion of patients in each stratum will be represented in the sample. In studies in general practice designed to measure the prevalence of disease, this approach will sometimes be appropriate in that the particular subject being studied may only be important in certain strata in the population, such as disability in the elderly, immunization status in children, or cervical cytology in women in the age group 20–65 years or hypertension in the age group 35–65 years. In some studies of the population designed to measure the incidence of disease where events occur with different frequency in different age, sex, or social class groups, it may also be helpful to draw samples of different sizes in different strata of the population. For instance, if events are common in one age group a one-in-five sample of that age group may be sufficient to provide meaningful results, while in another age group a one-in-two sample may be required. This approach may be appropriate in general practice in, for instance, studying the incidence of depression, strokes, or urinary tract infection, conditions which are markedly influenced by age and sex.

Other methods of sampling

When random sampling is not possible, systematic sampling may be carried out. For picking a one-in-eight systematic sample the simplest method is to take between one and eight a number at random as the starting point and then every eighth case record in the files should be sampled. Usually this results in a representative sample, but it is less certain than random sampling. Systematic sampling which depends on, for instance, the first letter of the patient's surname is never acceptable because it would inevitably group together patients in different cultural groups (such as the Jones and Patels). Year of birth has been suggested as a method of systematic sampling, but this carries with it risks of identifying groups of patients subjected to common seasonal or environmental hazards. A much more acceptable method of sampling is to use the date of birth in the month.

Non-response

In carrying out a sample survey, failure of individuals to respond to the survey is often a major problem. It is never possible to say whether the non-responders are a representative group of the total population, and if the non-response rate is high the results of the survey must be interpreted with caution.

In general practice surveys, non-response may be due to a variety of factors. General practice registers of patients are usually out-of-date. In some inner city practices up to 20 per cent of the population change address each year. If a sample is drawn from a practice register, it is likely to include a proportion of these patients. Very frequently the doctors in the practice know that a patient has left the district or died, but this information has not been transferred to the register. The first stage in sampling from a practice register should always be to present a list of the patients sampled to the partners and ask them to confirm that, to their knowledge, the patients are still registered with the practice at the address on the patient's record. If the survey consists of a postal contact with the patient, a proportion of letters will be returned by the post office, identifying that the patient has moved. If the survey is concerned with an interview, the interviewer may be able to identify patients who have moved out of the district. Finally, Family Practitioner Committees (FPCs) may be consulted to provide information about the patient's whereabouts, and Housing Departments can, on some occasions, be helpful.

Unfortunately there is no way of identifying patients who have moved into the practice area but have not registered for medical care and will not do so until they become ill. The practice is 'at risk' to these patients. In an area where there is a high level of population mobility they introduce an unavoidable error into any sampling method. In measuring demand for care those patients who register with the practice when they become ill are often considered to balance those who have left the area but are still registered with the practice. In measuring need by sampling and interview this assumption is not justified.

In carrying out random sample surveys in general practice it is important to ascertain that the patients in the sample are indeed still resident in the practice area and form part of the population being surveyed. If they do not, they can in some surveys be replaced by a further random sample. In surveys which are concerned with death or admission to hospital or an old people's home, however, it is important to retain them in the sample as this may be an important outcome measure.

In undertaking random sample surveys in general practice the following stages may therefore be carried out:

(1) draw a random sample from the practice register;
(2) check with the doctors in the practice that the patients in the sample are still registered with the practice;
(3) identify patients who cannot be contacted by the post office or personal visit;
(4) check all non-responders with the FPC;
(5) if acceptable to the particular study, replace non-responders by a further age/sex stratified random sample.

Confidence limits

The advantage of taking a random sample from the population of patients is that it makes it possible to calculate the probability that the average value or proportion measured in the sample accurately estimates the value of that variable in the population. In other words, using the sample size and the values recorded in the survey it is possible to state with some confidence the limits within which the true values in the population will lie. Thus if Dr Preston is concerned that there are many patients in his population who have undiagnosed hypertension, he may decide to measure the blood pressure of a random sample of 100 patients. If this reveals that 18 per cent have a diastolic blood pressure in excess of 110 mm of mercury, it is possible for him to predict with 95 per cent confidence that between 10 and 26 per cent of this population of patients have a blood pressure in excess of 110 mm of mercury. The way in which confidence limits are determined will be discussed in more detail in

Chapter 4. What is important at this stage is to recognize that random sampling, which depends on the rules of chance that each individual will have an equal opportunity of entering the sample, carries with it important statistical implications. As a result, if the doctor can provide an estimate of the proportion of patients in the practice likely to have a particular characteristic or disease, the statistician can advise on the size of the sample which must be studied to provide results which can be depended on within defined confidence limits.

STUDYING A RANDOM SAMPLE OF PATIENTS OVER THE AGE OF 65 YEARS

Dr Preston is impressed with the value of random sampling, but wonders what this implies for him in his practice if he decides to try to measure the amount of disability in his elderly population. His practice provides care for 10 000 patients and, of these, 952 are aged 65–74, and 670 are over the age of 75 years. The first problem he must deal with is that of describing clearly what he means by disability and what are the important disabilities he wishes to measure. In approaching this problem he must bear in mind that there is little point in identifying disabilities which cannot be reduced by the resources available. Dr Preston thinks that there are a lot of patients 'out there' who have remediable disabilities due to poor eyesight and poor hearing. He wants to try to assess the magnitude of these problems by studying a random sample of his patients over the age of 65 years.

He consults a statistician who asks him how many of the patients in this age group he expects to be suffering from these disabilities. This provides him with his first problem because he really has no idea, but suspects it is quite a lot. On the advice of the statistician he consults the literature and as a result is able to get some estimate of the prevalence of these problems. He estimates that each of these disabilities may be expected in about 20 per cent of the patients over the age of 65.

The statistician then asked Dr Preston how closely he hopes the measure of disability which he detects in his sample will reflect the probable true measure of disability in the population as a whole. Since he expects a level of each disability measured to be about 20 per cent, he would like to be able to infer from the results that the true value for the population is likely to be within plus or minus 5 per cent of the value detected in the study. To achieve this the statistician recommends that he should take a random sample of 222 patients over the age of 65.

The next problem is that of drawing a random sample. Dr Preston has an age/sex register in the practice, but patients do not have a unique practice number. He therefore decides that he will have to do the best he can and take a sequential sample starting with a random number and selecting every sixth patient over the age of 65 years. This will provide a sample size of 270 and allow for non-response of about 15 per cent.

Having identified this sample he must then define precisely the measurement he wishes to carry out. He is interested in disabilities and decides to define each of these in functional terms as follows:

(1) can the patient read the standard print of a newspaper with or without spectacles in normal daylight; and
(2) can the patient hear a normal conversational voice at a distance of eight feet?

His next problem is to decide who will carry out this survey and where it will take place. He would like the survey to be carried out in the patients' homes. He has three alternatives. The first is to persuade the attached health visitors to undertake the work. The second is to employ a part-time nurse in the practice and reclaim 70 per cent of her salary from the FPC. The third is to seek research funds to pay for a fieldworker to carry out the survey. The first alternative is not received with any enthusiasm by the health visitors. After a good deal of argument he persuades his partners that the employment of a part-time nurse is justified. The nurse is recruited to work five half-days per week. There are 270 patients to be visited. If each visit takes 30 minutes including travelling time, this represents about seven weeks' work.

However, time must be added on for re-visiting patients not at home on the first visit and for secretarial work. It would seem reasonable to employ the nurse for three months.

Clearly it is important to develop a system which will ensure that the work is carried out as efficiently as possible. The nurse draws the sample and for each patient in the sample prepares a record card. This includes the name, address, and, where available, the telephone number of the patient. She files these in alphabetical order and prepares a list of the patients in the sample for the partners to inspect. They are asked to identify any patients whom they know to have died or left the district. She then replaces these with a further random sample. She then prepares a letter for each of the partners to sign, addressed to their own patients, explaining the objectives of the survey and seeking the patient's co-operation. Some of these letters will be returned by the post office with 'Not known at this address' written on them. These patients can be replaced in the sample.

The nurse then develops a record which she will complete at each survey visit. This identifies the patient and includes the two main questions to be answered by the survey. It may be expanded to include other useful information, such as whether or not the patient is working, details of family resources, and other physical measurements. It is important, however, at this stage to ensure that any extra information collected is relevant to the study, and the temptation to collect extra information because it may be of some interest should be resisted. If further information is to be collected, it is important, as with the two primary questions, to define clearly what measurements are being made or what questions are being asked. Hopefully the final research record for each patient will not cover more than one side of a sheet of A4 paper.

The nurse is now ready to proceed with her survey. When possible she will telephone patients in advance of her visit, but some patients will not be on the telephone. She will zone her visits geographically to reduce travelling time, and at the end of each day will indicate on her card index the outcome of her work. A proportion of patients will not be at home when she visits and she will need to re-schedule these visits. A decision must be made as to how often she should re-visit before deciding that the patient is not accessible.

At the end of the survey it may be that 85 per cent of the sample have been visited and the record completed. It is then important to ensure that those who have been missed do not differ significantly in terms of age and sex from those who have been successfully visited. Extra information about the non-responders may be derived from the medical records and doubtless some will be found to be in full-time employment or to have visited the doctor during the period of the survey.

It should be decided in advance of the survey what action will be taken if abnormalities are identified. In this way it will be possible for the nurse to initiate action and explain this to the patient. In most cases this will be to arrange a visit to the doctor, in the first instance, who can then refine the diagnosis in terms of the disability identified and take appropriate action.

Was it worth it?

Doctor Preston now has a measure of visual and hearing disabilities in the elderly patients in his practice, which was the objective of his study, but he cannot help wondering if the patients in the sample have benefited from the study. He thinks the only way he can find this out is to re-measure the patients in the sample six months later, but then realizes that this will not be a reliable method of measuring the outcome of his survey because time is passing and his patients are developing more disabilities. He realizes that to answer this question he would need to compare his sample of patients with a control group. This he feels is in the field of the professional researcher. He did not, after all, set out to answer this question and is satisfied as a result of his survey that he knows the amount of disability due to visual and hearing loss in the patients in his practice, and he can now make a case to the health authority for the attachment of a health visitor for the elderly.

SCREENING AND CASE-FINDING

To study the size of a particular problem in his practice, Dr Preston has carried out a study of a sample of his patients. As a result of his findings he may decide that he should attempt to identify all patients in the practice with visual or hearing loss. This is described as screening; i.e. he visits the entire population of interest or invites them to attend the practice for a particular test or investigation.

Wilson and Jungner (1968) drew up a series of criteria which should be met before a population is submitted to pre-symptomatic screening. These criteria have stood the test of time and are useful guidelines:

(1) the condition should be important;
(2) an accepted treatment must be available for the condition;
(3) the facilities for diagnosis and treatment must be available;
(4) a latent or early presymptomatic stage in the condition must exist;
(5) a suitable screening test must be available;
(6) the test/examination must be acceptable to the population;
(7) the natural history of the condition must be understood;
(8) an agreed treatment policy on whom to treat must exist;
(9) the cost must be acceptable;
(10) surveying must be a continuing process and not a once-for-all project.

The criteria hold good for screening in general practice populations as in wider population screening. Although they were originally designed to guide those concerned with pre-symptomatic screening, many of the criteria are equally applicable for screening for established disability; for example, criteria 1–3 and 6–9. In general practice, however, patients are seen at regular intervals by their doctor, and if he wishes, for instance, to identify all the patients in his practice with, say, visual disability or an abnormal blood pressure, he can achieve this, probably more economically, simply by recording the vision or blood pressure of patients who attend. It has been demonstrated that about 93 per cent of patients attend the general practitioner at least once in every five years (Holland *et al.* 1977). In a screening survey in general practice it was demonstrated that in the context of hypertension all the patients found on screening to have a blood pressure in excess of 115 mm of mercury diastolic had been seen by the doctor within this period of time (D'Souza *et al.* 1976). This method of identifying pre-symptomatic disease in general practice has been described as 'case-finding' (Sackett and Holland 1975).

For those individuals in the population who visit the general practitioner at fairly regular intervals this is almost certainly the most cost-effective way of identifying asymptomatic disease. Other methods depend on the doctor inviting the patient to attend for a particular test, and it is well known that up to 50 per cent fail to respond to such an invitation, or visiting patients in their homes, which is very expensive.

Case-finding, however, does demand a major change in the attitude of general practitioners to their preventive role and it demands more time for booked consultations in general practice. It also demands a more disciplined approach to medical recording. If it is to be achieved the doctor must include in his medical records a prominent place for recording important examinations. This alerts him at each consultation if these examinations have not been carried out and recorded.

It is doubtful whether general practitioners, trained in the main to respond to new symptoms of illness, are currently sufficiently aware of their preventive role to undertake effective case-finding, and this was clearly a problem which was faced by Dr Preston. If, however, case-finding is regarded as an important function of general practitioners in identifying their patients' needs, it is necessary to support the doctors with clerical help. Constant supervision of the doctors' performance is required, which almost certainly means that the records should be reviewed at a proportion of the consulting sessions by a clerical assistant who can record and feed-back to the doctors their performance. The clerical supervision is likely to produce benefits which outweigh any costs in terms of identifying pre-symptomatic disease or disability.

With good case-finding in general practice there will still be certain segments of the population in which surveys must be carried out. This applies particularly to the very elderly and housebound. These patients may not be able to consult the doctor or may regard their disabilities as due simply to age and not appropriate for medical care. In this age group such disabilities as deterioration in vision and hearing and problems with locomotion are particularly important and, in some cases, major disabilities produced by, for instance, heart failure, as Dr Preston discovered, may be identified.

REFERENCES

Banks, M., Beresford, S., Morrell, D. C., Watkins, C. J., and Waller, J. (1975). Factors influencing demand for primary medical care in women aged 20–44 years. *International Journal of Epidemiology* **4,** 189–95.

Bergner, H., Bobbett, R. A., Carter, W. B., and Gibson, B. S. (1981). The Sickness Impact Profile; development and final reviews of a health status measure. *Medical Care* **19,** 787–805.

D'Souza, M., Swan, A., and Shannon, D. (1976). A longterm controlled trial of screening in general practice. *Lancet* **1,** 1228–31.

Dunnell, K. and Cartwright, A. (1972). Medical takers, prescribers and hoarders. Routledge and Kegan Paul, Andover, Hants.

Goldberg, D. (1972) *The detection of psychiatric illness by questionnaire.* Maudsley Monograph 21. Oxford University Press, Oxford.

Holland, W., Creese, A., D'Souza, M., *et al.* (1977). A controlled trial of multiphasic screening in middle age. *International Journal of Epidemiology* **6,** 350–63.

Hunt, S., McEwen, J., and McKenna, S. P. (1985). Measuring health status: a new tool for clinicians and epidemiologists. *Journal of Royal College of General Practitioners* **35,** 185–8.

MRC (Medical Research Council) (1960). Standardized questionnaire on respiratory symptoms. *British Medical Journal* **2,** 1665.

Sackett, D. and Holland, W. (1975). Controversy in the detection of disease. *Lancet* **2,** 357–9.

Wilson, J. and Jungner, G. (1968). *Principles and practice of screening for disease.* World Health Organization, Geneva.

4 Is it normal?

Martin Roland

Dr Preston lay awake after visiting his patient who had been having an acute attack of asthma. Life certainly had seemed easier when he was a trainee. Was it normal—he wondered—to see 50 patients in a day? One Monday, shortly after he came, he had seen 58 patients in surgery and done seven home visits. The parents of the asthmatic child said that she had been getting worse for two days—but they thought it was normal. He thought of the patients in his morning surgery—how could he decide whether the 50-year-old's blood pressure was normal or whether the spinster's serum potassium of 3.3 mol/l was normal? He remembered that the statistics book he had glanced at for the exam for Membership of the Royal College of General Practitioners had said something about 'Normality'—and then he fell asleep.

WHAT DOES A STATISTICIAN MEAN BY 'NORMAL'?

One of the characteristics of people is the marked variation that occurs between individuals. For example, the average height of a British man is 5′7″, but one fairly frequently sees men from 5′2″ up to 6′1″. Another example is the consultation rate—people on average consult their general practitioner about three times a year, but there are a few people in every practice who hardly ever see a doctor, and a few who are in and out of the surgery every week.

A frequency distribution may be shown by a table which consists of all values which can be taken by a variable (e.g. height, number of consultations per year) and which shows the frequency with which each of these values occur. Statisticians often describe a series of observations or a frequency distribution as being 'Normally distributed'. A typical 'Normal' distribution —height of British men—is shown in Fig. 4.1. The characteristics of a Normal distribution are that it is bell-shaped and symmetrical about its middle point. A frequency distribution which has a long tail in one direction is called skew. Figure 4.2 shows an example of a skew distribution—the amount of time spent with the patient in a series of general practice consultations. In this example, most patients spend between two and eight minutes with the doctor, but a few are seen for 20 minutes or longer. This distribution is certainly not symmetrical about its middle point.

The Normal distribution is a mathematical idealization of a distribution which is uncommonly found in biological work. However, many statistical tests require the assumption that the readings are Normally distributed. Statisticians

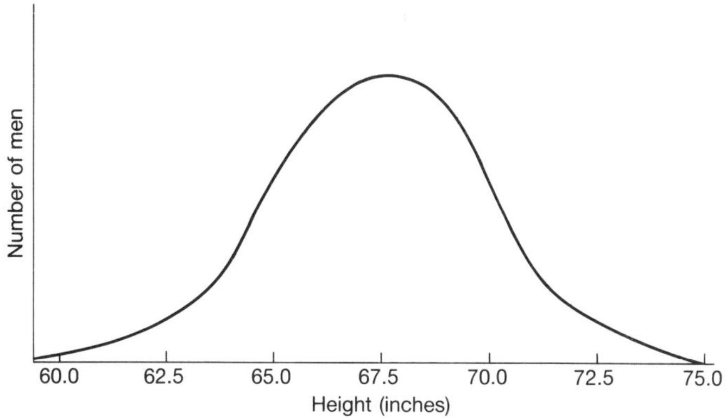

Fig. 4.1. A Normal distribution—height of adult men.

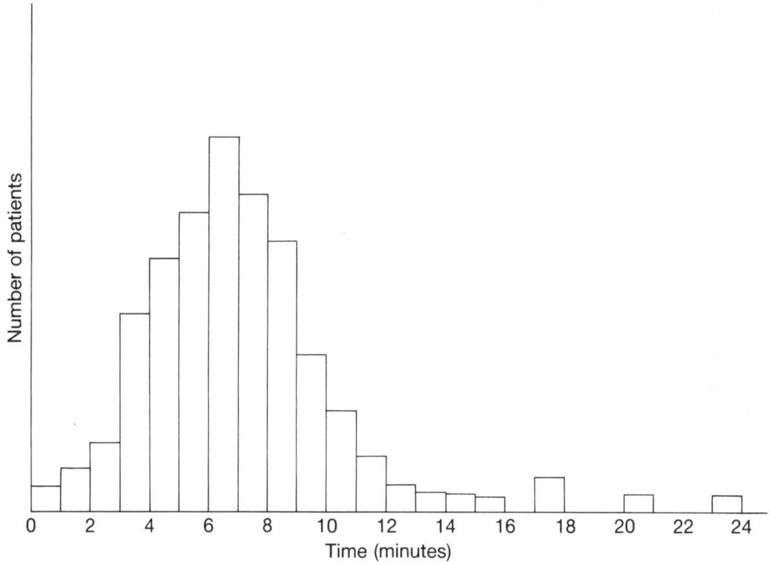

Fig. 4.2. A skew distribution—time spent with patients in consultations.

therefore like readings to be Normally distributed as this increases the range and power of analytical methods available to them. If the distribution of readings is approximately Normal, it is still possible to use these tests. Often it is possible to make the data conform more closely to a Normal distribution by using the logarithm of a set of readings in the analysis—this technique is called transformation. If the distribution of a set of readings cannot be approximated to Normal by this method, then the data are usually analysed by one of a number of 'non-parametric' tests. These tests, which include, for example, the

Mann–Whitney U test and the Wilcoxon signed rank test, do not require the assumption that data are Normally distributed. They are described in more detail in the statistical textbooks listed at the end of the chapter.

The characteristics of a Normal distribution are determined entirely by the middle point—or average—and by the variability or scatter, so these are now described in more detail.

Measures of position—the average

There are three commonly used ways of working out average values. In a series of observations, the mode is the value which is found to occur most frequently. The mean—often called the average—is the sum of all the measurements divided by the number of measurements. The median is the observation or measurement lying in the middle when the observations are listed in increasing order—so there are an equal number of observations which are larger and smaller than the median. If there are an even number of observations (say 20), the median is the point midway between the two middle readings (the 10th and 11th in a series of 20 readings).

In a Normal distribution, the mode, mean, and median all have the same value—at the peak of the bell-shaped curve. In a skewed distribution, they may all have different values (Fig. 4.3). In this example the number of consultations found most frequently (the mode) is one consultation per year. Because the distribution is skewed by a few patients who consult 30 or even 35 times per year, the mean value is more than twice as large as the mode. However, even in a series of readings which is approximately normally distributed, the mean is rarely enough to describe a series of observations. Some measure needs to be given of the spread of observations around the central point.

Measures of spread—the standard deviation

The standard deviation describes the spread of a distribution. For Normally distributed data, approximately two-thirds of observations fall within one standard deviation of the mean, and 95 per cent of observations fall within two standard deviations of the mean (Fig. 4.4).

The formula for calculating the standard deviation is shown below. Many basic calculators will do the job automatically.

Formula for calculating standard deviation

The standard deviation (SD) can be calculated from the formula:

$$\sqrt{\left(\Sigma\frac{(x^2)-(\sum x)^2/n}{n-1}\right)}$$

where $\sum x$ represents the sum of all the observations

$\sum x^2$ represents the observations each squared, then added up, and

n represents the number of observations.

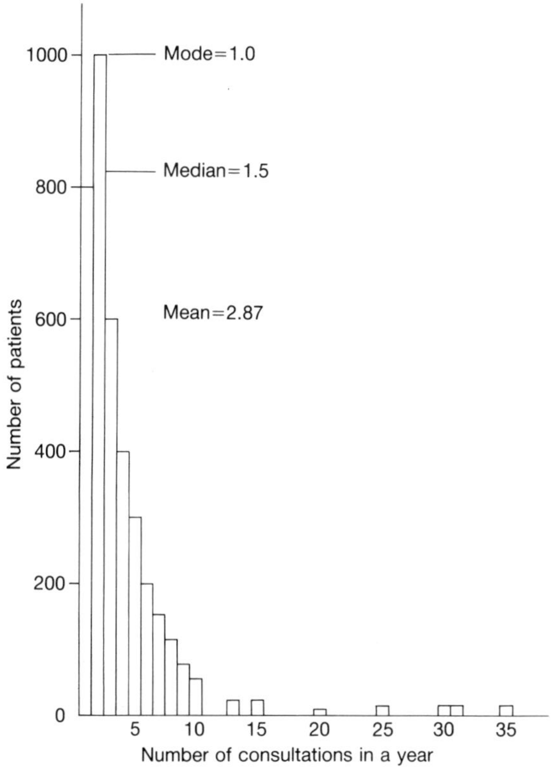

Fig. 4.3. Mode, median, and mean in a skew distribution.

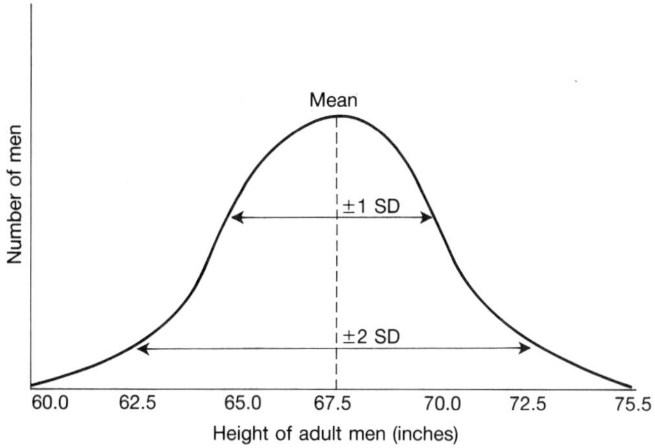

Fig. 4.4. Distribution of height of adult men.

Example of standard deviation calculation

During the first half of 1986, the numbers of patients that Dr Preston saw in surgery each week were 120, 154, 133, 162, 145, 108. What are the mean and standard deviation?

$$\text{Mean} = \frac{120+154+133+161+145+108}{6} = \frac{882}{6} = 136$$

Standard deviation:

$$\textstyle\sum x \quad = 822; \ (\sum x)^2 = 822 \times 822 = 675\,684$$

$$\textstyle\sum(x^2) = 120^2 + 154^2 + 133^2 + 162^2 + 145^2 + 108^2 = 114\,738$$

$$\text{Standard deviation} = \sqrt{\left(\frac{114\,738 - 675\,684/6}{5}\right)} = 20.5.$$

The standard deviation is often quoted in papers as a measure of spread. However, the theory that about 95 per cent of observations fall within two standard deviations of the mean only applies to Normal distributions. If this theory is used on a skew distribution, the result may be nonsense. For example, in Fig. 4.3 the mean number of consultations is 2.82 per year. The standard deviation is 2.9. This implies that in two thirds of cases the number of consultations ought to be in the range from −0.8 to 5.72 consultations per year. This is clearly nonsense as there cannot be a negative number of consultations in a year. Statements about the standard deviation may be misleading if the data are clearly not Normally distributed.

A better measure of spread for a skew distribution is the interquartile range—which is the range from the value below which one-quarter of the observations lie to the value above which one-quarter of the observations lie.

There are two main reasons for wanting to know the standard deviation:

(1) it is needed for a number of statistical tests which compare the mean value of one group of observations with the mean value of another—e.g. the *t*-test;
(2) it is used to calculate confidence intervals.

Confidence intervals

Having found one woman with a serum potassium of 3.3 mmol/l, Dr Preston decided to measure the serum potassium of the next two patients whom he saw on diuretics—those readings were 4.0 mmol/l and 4.7 mmol/l, so the mean of the three values was 4.0 mmol/l. He could have concluded that the average serum potassium of patients on diuretics was 4.0 mmol/l, but three patients is a pretty small sample, so he might well have been wrong. He therefore decided to measure the serum potassium of the next 50 patients whom he saw on diuretics. Now the mean value of serum potassium for these 50 patients would not necessarily be the same as that for another group of 50 patients on diuretics. However, the more patients that Dr Preston includes in his sample the more likely it is that the results will approximate to the true population mean serum potassium for all patients on diuretics.

This example illustrates what is meant by 'sampling error'. In most medical research, observations are made on a sample of patients with a given condition rather than on the whole population of such patients. Calculating confidence limits for readings which have been obtained on a sample of patients allows one to generalize the results to the population at large. If the sample is very small, then the confidence limits will be very wide, and vice versa.

Calculating confidence limits for a mean value shows the likely error that may have arisen in estimating the mean value on that sample. If one calculates the 95 per cent confidence limits for a mean value, those are the limits within which one can be 95 per cent sure that the true mean value lies. An approximate formula for calculating confidence limits is:

$$95\%\ \text{confidence limits} = \text{mean} \pm \left(2 \times \frac{\text{standard deviation}}{\sqrt{(\text{number of observations})}}\right)$$

If Dr Preston measured the mean serum potassium on 50 patients as 4.2 mmol/l with a standard deviation of 0.5 mmol/l, he can be 95 per cent certain that the mean serum potassium for patients on diuretics lies between 4.06 and 4.34 mmol/l:

$$95\%\ \text{confidence limits} = 4.2 \pm \left(2 \times \frac{0.5}{\sqrt{50}}\right)$$

$$= 4.2 \pm 0.14$$

$$= 4.06\text{–}4.34\ \text{mmol/l.}$$

Confidence intervals can also be calculated for proportions. When Dr Preston is on call at weekends, he also covers for the patients of another practice of similar size. The calls always seem to come from the other practice, so he decides to keep a tally. Over five weekends on call, he had 100 calls. Forty of these are from his own practice (40 per cent) and 60 from the other practice (60 per cent). By calculating the confidence limits, he can work out within what limits the proportion of visits arising from the other practice would be likely to lie if he went on recording for a much longer period of time. An approximate formula for the 95 per cent confidence limits of a proportion (p) is:

$$95\%\ \text{confidence limits} = p \pm \left[2 \times \sqrt{\left(\frac{p \times (1-p)}{n}\right)}\right]$$

where n is the number of observations.

In this example, p is the proportion of calls arising from the other practice

(0.60) and *n* is the number of visits (100). Applying these figures to the formula gives:

$$
\begin{aligned}
95\%\ \text{confidence limits} &= 0.06 \pm \left[2 \times \sqrt{\left(\frac{(0.60 \times 0.40)}{100}\right)}\right] \\
&= 0.60 \pm 0.098 \\
&= 0.502\text{–}0.698.
\end{aligned}
$$

The 95 per cent confidence limits (0.502–0.698) for the proportion of visits arising from the other practice show that he can be fairly sure that his hunch about the other practice's calls was right: if he collected data on a larger sample of visits, he would almost certainly confirm that the other practice was responsible for more than 50 per cent of the calls.

Confidence limits give much more information about the distribution of a set of values than the standard deviation. Furthermore, confidence limits can be calculated on data which is not statistically 'Normal'. The *British Medical Journal* (Langman 1986) now requires authors to include confidence limits where appropriate in papers submitted for publication.

WHAT ELSE IS MEANT BY 'NORMAL'?

The Normal distribution, as defined by statisticians, is useful because it leads to the calculation of confidence limits and allows the use of many statistical tests. In practice, however, the word Normal is often used in other ways, as described next.

'*I thought it was normal, doctor*'

Much of the time the common meanings of the word normal are socially defined. These definitions are often dependent on the health beliefs and expectations of individuals—which may vary widely. A 70-year-old with treatable congestive cardiac failure may regard her breathlessness as 'normal' because it is what she has become used to over many months. Likewise, an 80-year-old man may regard deafness as 'normal' and not bother to ask his doctor whether the situation could be improved by removing wax or supplying a hearing aid.

At the other extreme the normally increased menstrual loss of a depressed perimenopausal woman may be presented as 'flooding' and urgent action demanded. The general practitioner in his surgery is constantly comparing symptoms presented by patients with his own perceptions of the acceptable range of human physiology and behaviour.

'*Your baby's weight is normal*'

The doctor may mean that the weight lies within the 90th centile on a growth chart, or he may mean that the baby is continuing to gain weight along a particular centile line. Figure 4.5 shows a centile chart for infants' weight. The baby whose growth is plotted on line A is light (on the 3rd centile line), but is growing normally because the line of weight gain is parallel to the 3rd centile line. The baby whose growth is plotted on line B might cause more concern. The weight of this baby was initially on the 90th centile line, but at the age of 12 months the growth rate appears suddenly to have reduced. The weight gain of this baby is not normal despite the fact that he is heavier at every age than the baby whose growth is shown in line A.

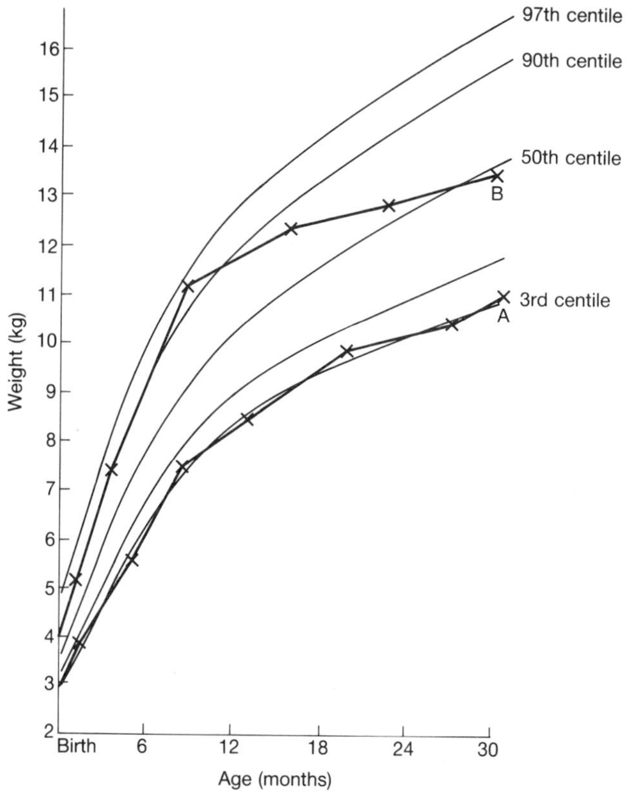

Fig. 4.5. Centile chart for a baby boy's weight (see text for explanation).

'Your blood pressure is normal'

In this example the word 'normal' has a clear meaning in relation to prognosis. The doctor knows from epidemiological studies and from clinical trials that, for example, a middle-aged man with a diastolic blood pressure of over 110 mm Hg is at greatly increased risk of developing a cerebro-vascular accident in the following 10 years, and he knows that treatment of that degree of hypertension is associated with a reduction in the risk. Therefore, when reassuring the patient about his blood pressure, he is thinking in terms of prognosis, and regards the patient as having 'no additional risk of cardiovascular or cerebro-vascular disease'.

'*Your cervical smear is normal*'

In this example, the doctor attempts to distinguish in a clear-cut way between normal and abnormal smears. In this context the word 'normal' has a meaning in relation both to prognosis and to diagnosis. When the doctor says 'Your smear is normal', he means 'You have a very low risk of developing cancer of the cervix between now and your next smear in three years time'. The doctor is also aware that the smear result is not just 'normal' or 'abnormal'. The result is graded, so that 'mild dysplasia' indicates a relatively low probability of developing carcinoma of the cervix over three years, whereas 'carcinoma *insitu*' indicates a high probability of invasive cancer developing.

In using the word 'normal' in relation to clinical tests, the doctor is no longer talking about biological variability in the healthy population, but is concerned with the predictive value of a diagnostic test in terms of prognosis for that patient.

Interpreting the results of tests

Diagnostic tests are never 100 per cent accurate. There may be false positives—where the test result is abnormal in a patient who does not really have the disease, and false negatives—where the test result is normal in a patient who has the disease. An example of the way in which a normal or abnormal test result contributes to the diagnosis of a disease is seen in Table 4.1, which shows some hypothetical figures for the predictive value of an electrocardiogram (ECG) in 100 patients presenting to a general practitioner with acute chest pain. The terms sensitivity and specificity (Table 4.2) are sometimes used with information of this type. The sensitivity of a test is the percentage of those with the disease who have a positive test result— i.e. 8/10 = 80 per cent in the example in Table 4.1. The specificity is the percentage of those without the disease who have a normal test result—i.e. 80/90 = 89 per cent in the example in Table 4.1. These terms often get muddled up. One way to get them the right way round is to remember that the sensitivity of a test reflects its ability to identify those who are sick, i.e have the disease (sen**S**itivity—**S**ick), while the specificity shows how good the test is at identifying those who are fit (speci**F**icity—**F**it).

For diseases with a low probability (e.g. myocardial infarction in patients presenting to general practitioners with chest pain), these terms can be misleading. In this situation it is more useful to calculate the precentage of positives that are true positives—8/18 = 44 per cent in the example. This is called the positive predictive value of the test. The negative predictive value is

Table 4.1. *Predictive value of ECG in chest pain (hypothetical figures)*

ECG result	MI† subsequently confirmed	MI† subsequently not confirmed	Totals
Ischaemia or infarction	8	10	18
Normal	2	80	82
Totals	10	90	100

†Myocardial infarction.

Table 4.2. *Predictive value of diagnostic tests*

Test result	Disease present	Disease absent
Positive	*a* (true positives	*b* (false positives)
Negative	*c* (false negatives)	*d* (true negatives)

% false positive $= [b/(a+b)] \times 100$
%false negative $= [c/(c+d)] \times 100$
Positive predictive value (%) $= [a/(a+b)] \times 100$
Negative predictive value (%) $= [d/(c+d)] \times 100$
Sensitivity $= a/(a+c)$
Specificity $= d/(b+d)$

the percentage of negatives which are true negatives (98 per cent).

The value of a diagnostic test will depend to a large extent on how much overlap there is between the results of the test for those who do and for those who do not have the disorder in question. In hypothyroidism, for example, the predictive value of serum cholesterol is low, as many patients with raised serum cholesterol do not have myxoedema. A raised plasma thyroid stimulating hormone (TSH), on the other hand, has a very high predictive value: almost all patients with raised TSH will have hypothyroidism.

Test results and clinical decisions

Knowledge of a test result influences the decisions taken by a doctor, because the test result alters the probability that a disease is present or absent. For example, using the hypothetical figures from Table 4.1, the overall probability of a patient presenting to his general practioner with chest pain having had a myocardial infarction is 10/100 (= 10 per cent). If, however, the ECG is normal, the probability of the patient having a myocardial infarction is reduced to 2/82 (= 2.4 per cent). The normal ECG does not exclude a myocardial infarction, but in this example the information given by a normal

ECG reduces the probability of the patient having had a myocardial infarction by a factor of four.

If a number of tests are carried out the combined contribution of the tests to the probability of a disease being present may be computed using a mathematical theory called Bayes' theorem. Bayes' theorem is the basis of some computer programs which have been developed to aid medical diagnosis. In an evaluation of the contribution of one such program to the diagnosis of acute abdominal pain, processing of information on symptoms, signs, and diagnostic tests by a computer was found to improve the initial diagnostic accuracy from 46 per cent to 65 per cent, and to reduce the negative laparotomy rate from 25 per cent to 10 per cent (Adams *et al.* 1986).

Reliability

A further aspect of any test or observation which is important in interpreting the results is the reliability of the test. Reliability—sometimes called repeatability—is the extent to which the test or observation gives the same result when done twice under the same conditions.

Measurement of blood urea level is a very reliable test. If it is done on two occasions, a week apart, the results will almost certainly be very similar, as laboratories exercise strict quality control over the test machinery. Blood urea is not subject to much biological variation, so change in a patient's blood urea from 5 mmol/l to 10 mmol/l would be likely to reflect a real change in his condition. Blood sugar level is also a reliable measure when done in the laboratory: if a specimen of blood in a fluoride tube is analysed twice in the laboratory, the results will be very similar. If the same sample is analysed twice using a blood glucose 'stick' test, then the agreement between the two readings will be less close—the 'stick' test is less reliable. However, blood glucose is also subject to much greater biological variation than blood urea. One measurement of blood urea will normally be sufficient to describe whether a patient is in renal failure, but a series of measurements may be needed to decide how good a patient's blood glucose control is.

Muscle spasm, on the other hand, is a very unreliable measurement in patients with acute back pain. There are no instruments which will give 'readings' of muscle spasm, and the amount of spasm may vary from minute to minute depending on the position which the patient is trying to adopt.

When reading published research it is important to look to see whether the authors have considered the reliability of their observations. If more than two observers have been involved, have they checked to see that they are recording in a standardized way?

CONCLUSION

Statistical concepts of normality are important to the doctor when he interprets the results of a test which he has arranged and when he reads and interprets published data. The calculation of confidence limits, which arises from the theory of the normal distribution, is particularly important in allowing him to generalize from the results of a sample of observations. This is very relevant to the general practitioner who wants to review some aspect of his own work—for example, records of the smoking history or cervical cytology status of his patients—but does not have the resources to examine the notes of all the relevant patients. By taking a sample he will be able to make an estimate of the quantity in which he is interested.

General practitioners continually use concepts of normal behaviour in their working lives. They often see diseases early in their natural history and are called on to decide whether a particular set of symptoms and signs is normal or whether the probability of a disease being present is sufficient to ask the patient to return for a further consultation or for a diagnostic test. The change of the patient's symptom with time or the result of a diagnostic test may influence the general practitioner's subsequent management decisions.

The general practitioner's assessment of what is normal for a particular patient will be influenced by his preceding knowledge about the patient. So, if Mrs Jones, who is forever in the surgery, consults with a lump in her throat, he may well decide that the probability of the symptoms being due to an ear, nose, and throat malignancy is extremely small and choose to ignore it. On the other hand, if Mr Brown, who has hardly consulted in the past 20 years, came with the same complaint he might judge that the symptom reporting was outside Mr Brown's normal range of behaviour and arrange an urgent barium swallow.

The general practitioner who becomes skilled in diagnosis will have an appreciation of the range of normal behaviour, a knowledge of the relative probability of individual disease states occurring, and he will have learnt to apply this knowledge to the problem presented by an individual patient.

FURTHER READING

Armitage, P. (1971). *Statistical methods in medical research*. Blackwell Scientific Publications, Oxford. (A more advanced statistical textbook, which requires an understanding of algebraic notation.)

Bradford Hill, A. (1984). *Short textbook of medical statistics*. Hodder and Stoughton, Sevenoaks, Kent. (Good descriptive style for basic statistics.)

Gore, S. M. and Attman, D. G. (1982). *Statistics in practice*. British Medical Association, London. (Particularly good sections on how to interpret published research, especially clinical trials.)

Sackett, D. L., Haynes, R. B., and Tugwell, P. (1985). *Clinical epidemiology—a basic science for clinical medicine*. Little Brown, Boston, Mass. (Good sections on interpreting diagnostic tests.)

REFERENCES

Adams, I. D., Chan, M., Clifford, P. C., *et al.* (1986). Computer aided diagnosis of acute abdominal pain: a multicentre study. *British Medical Journal* **293,** 800–4.

Langman, M. J. S. (1986). Towards estimation and confidence intervals. *British Medical Journal* **292,** 716.

5 Is it significant—is it important?

Martin Roland

'. . . and women who had been oral contraceptive users were significantly more likely to develop breast cancer ($p < 0.01$)'. Dr Preston sighed as he put down the journal. What did it mean? Should he be taking long-term users off the pill? He knew these results conflicted with those of a number of other studies. And what of the significance level? Did that mean the result was important?

WHAT DOES 'STATISTICALLY SIGNIFICANT' MEAN?

It is usual in most sorts of research or audit to study a sample of the patients in whom the researcher is interested. Thus, for example, studies of the pill and breast cancer do not look at all patients on the pill, or at all patients with breast cancer. Observations are made on a sample of patients, which is chosen in such a way that the results can hopefully be generalized to the larger group (e.g. all women on the pill).

The main disadvantage of using samples is that some precision is lost. For instance, if the incidence of breast cancer was examined in two groups of 1000 women, the first group born on odd days of the month (e.g. 7/8/51) and the second group on even days of the months (e.g. 8/8/51), one would not expect any systematic difference between the groups, but the incidence of breast cancer in the two groups might be different by chance. The difference in measurements made on two samples which may be due to chance is called 'sampling error'.

The lack of precision in a measurement on a sample is expressed in terms of confidence intervals, which were described in Chapter 4. If a measurement is made on a very small sample, it will be imprecise and the confidence intervals will be wide. If the measurement is made on a large sample, it will be a precise estimate of the value in a large population, and the confidence intervals will be small. The size of the confidence interval relates to the size of the sampling error which is likely to have been present in the measurement.

Significance tests relate to *differences* in measurements which have been made on two samples; for example, the incidence of breast cancer in women on the pill compared to diaphragm users. The word significant, when used in the statistical sense, means 'not easily explained by sampling error', which is sometimes phrased 'not due to chance'. If a statistical test shows that a difference between two measurements is significant at the 5 per cent level

($p<0.05$), this means that there is a 95 per cent chance that the difference is genuine, and only a 5 per cent chance that the observed difference is due to chance, or sampling error. If a difference is significant at the 1 per cent level ($p<0.01$), there is a 99 per cent chance that the difference is genuine, and only a 1 per cent chance that the observed difference is due to sampling error.

Although a test of statistical significance indicates how likely it is that an observed difference between two sets of measurements is due to chance, it does not tell whether that difference is of clinical significance. A result may be statistically significant without being of clinical significance or importance. Likewise, a result may not be statistically significant, but may be of considerable clinical importance. The following examples illustrate ways in which these situtions may arise.

RESULT STATISTICALLY SIGNIFICANT, BUT NOT CLINICALLY IMPORTANT

Actual differences small

If a sample is very large, then quite small differences may reach clinical significance. Table 5.1 shows some hypothetical figures for the response of 1000 patients with sore throat to penicillin or placebo. Of the 500 who received penicillin, 450 (90 per cent) were symptom-free within five days, compared to 435 (87 per cent) in the placebo group. This difference is clearly not of any great clinical significance, but the difference is statistically significant—the probability of this difference having arisen by chance is only 2 per cent.

Table 5.1. *Example of difference which is statistically significant but clinically unimportant in the case of sore throat treatment*

	Treatment	
Outcome after five days	Penicillin	Placebo
Still symptomatic	50	65
Symptom-free	450	435
Totals	500	500
	$\chi_1^2=5.2$; $p=0.02$	

When looking at the results of a research study, do not just look at the significance level, look at the actual difference which has to be shown to see whether the result looks to be of clinical significance as well as statistical significance.

Inappropriate comparisons

Table 5.2 shows the proportion of *Escherichia coli* resistant to ampicillin in patients with urinary infection. In the Aberdeen study, 50 per cent of *E. coli* were resistant to ampicillin, compared to only 10 per cent in the Bristol study—a difference which is highly statistically significant ($p<0.001$). Can one conclude that there is more antibiotic resistance in Scotland than England?

Table 5.2. *Example is statistically significant, but comparison is invalid*

	Aberdeen (100 hospital in-patients)	Bristol (100 general practice patients)
E. coli in urine resistant to ampicillin (%)	50	10
E. coli in urine sensitive to ampicillin (%)	50	90
Totals	100	100
	$\chi_1^2=36.2$; $p<0.001$	

This would be a false conclusion, as the Aberdeen patients were hospital in-patients and the Bristol patients were recruited from general practice. It is well known that a much greater proportion of bacteria isolated in hospital are resistant to antibiotics compared to those isolated in general practice. The difference is probably nothing to do with the different geographical locations of the studies. The observed geographical difference is statistically significant, but not clinically relevant as it is based on an invalid comparison. If the design of a study is incorrect or if a comparison is inappropriate, statistical manipulation of the data will not produce meaningful results.

Problem of non-responders

In a study on the effectiveness of an educational booklet for patients with back pain, the booklet was given at random to half of a group of patients with back pain. One month later, a questionnaire was sent, testing the patients' knowledge about back pain to see whether they had learned anything from the booklet (Table 5.3). The knowledge scores of those who had received the booklet were significantly greater than that of the control group. Does this mean that the patients who had received the booklet actually had learned more about back pain? This may be true, but it is not a conclusion that can be drawn from this study. Look at the return rate in Table 5.3. Only half the 'booklet' group returned their questionnaires! What of the other half? They are likely to be less well educated and motivated than those who did return their questionnaires—there may even have been some illiterate patients in this group. The response rate to the questionnaire is so poor, and may have been biased in favour of the more educated, so it is really not possible to draw conclusions about the group as a whole.

Table 5.3. *Example is statistically significant, but invalid because of poor response rate*

	Given educational booklet	Not given educational booklet (controls)
Number in original group	50	50
Number returning questionnaire	25	35
Mean score of knowledge about back pain (standard deviation)	24(8)	18(6)

Difference in knowledge scores is statistically significant ($t_{58}=3.3$; $p < 0.01$)

Repeated significance testing

Conventionally, a result is regarded as being statistically significant if the probability that the result is due to sampling error is less than 5 per cent. However, this applies to each test which is done. If 20 significance tests are done, one would expect one to show a positive result on the basis of chance alone.

In a study of referral behaviour, data were collected on one week's workload from 20 doctors. In the course of the analysis the hypothesis was tested that more patients are referred to hospital from Friday evening surgeries. For 19 of the doctors there seemed to be no relationship between referral pattern and day of the week. However, one doctor referred more patients on Friday evening, and the effect was statistically significant at the 5 per cent level. Can one conclude that this doctor has a particular pattern of pre-weekend behaviour? No. The conclusion might be invalid. Individual statistical tests have been performed on data from each of the 20 doctors. On the basis of chance alone, one could expect one of the analyses to have been significant at the 5 per cent level.

Beware of studies where many individual statistical tests seem to have been performed. If multiple tests have been done, it is safer only to accept those results which are significant at the 1 per cent level ($p<0.01$).

These examples show situations where a result is statistically significant, but is of little or no clinical relevance. There are also situations where a result could be clinically important, but is not statistically significant.

RESULT POSSIBLY IMPORTANT, BUT NOT STATISTICALLY SIGNIFICANT

Sample size too small

Table 5.4 shows the hypothetical results of a trial in which patients on regular tranquillizers were randomly assigned to continued conventional management or to a tranquillizer support group. After 16 weeks, two-thirds of those attending the tranquillizer support group have come off tranquillizers, compared to only one-third in the conventional management group. This clearly could be an important difference—the support group appears to double the chance of coming off tranquillizers, but the result is not statistically significant. This experimentdoes not adequately answer the question of which method of tranquillizer withdrawal is best. The apparent differences between the two methods would be worth investigating further with a larger sample. This would clarify whether the difference observed in this study was due to a true difference between the methods or whether it was due to sampling error. If the number of patients in the trial of the tranquillizer support group had been twice as large, the difference between the two groups would have been statistically significant, even if the proportion giving up tranquillizers were the same as in the example.

When reading the results of a research study, do not just look at the significance level. Look at the actual values. If the results look important, maybe the sample was too small for statistical significance to be reached.

Table 5.4. *Clinically important results which are not statistically significant*

	Tranquillizer support group	Conventional management
Number still taking tranquillizers after 16 weeks	5	10
Number who have stopped tranquillizers after 16 weeks	10	5

$\chi_1^2 = 2.13$; $p = 0.14$

Problems of accurate data collection

Ideally, the doctor who is doing research, or the doctor who is looking at some aspect of his own work, wants to base conclusions on reliable information. However, it is often difficult to collect reliable information about problems which are important to general practitioners. Table 5.5 gives a list of the sort of things which general practitioners may want to collect information about, along with some of the difficulties which they may encounter.

Inaccuracies which occur in data collection may be sufficiently large to obscure an important effect. For instance, if Dr Preston wanted to compare the consultation rate in the old established part of his practice with that in a

Table 5.5. *Examples of problems in data collection*

Information sought	Problem
Retrospective data from notes	Incomplete records, e.g. prescriptions or visits not entered
Patient satisfaction	Patients do not like to criticize their doctor, so are reluctant to complain
Sickness absence	Patients only need a certificate for more than a week off work—difficult to measure repeated short absence
Individual list size in partnerships	Number of patients for whom a doctor effectively provides care is often not the same as nominal list size

new housing estate, he would be in great difficulty if he knew that one of his partners, who happened to look after the new housing estate, frequently saw patients without making any entry in the medical records. The information which he could extract from the notes under these circumstances would be seriously flawed, and he might well fail to demonstrate a genuinely increased consultation rate for those patients living in the housing estate.

The well-known adage 'garbage in, garbage out' is true. No amount of statistical manipulation will salvage data which is inherently flawed.

'Are these results important?'

The examples given above show that there is a considerable difference between clinical significance or importance and statistical significance. Life for the busy general practitioner reading journals would be much easier if statistical significance indicated a result which was important to him, but that does not necessarily follow.

Here are some of the questions that Dr Preston could ask himself as he reads journal articles. They will help him sort out the important results from those that are only significant in a statistical sense. These points are discussed in more detail in the reference books listed at the end of the chapter.

1. Read the summary. If the results were valid, would they be useful to you? If so, read on.
2. Were patients in the study similar to the patients you are likely to meet in practice?
3. Have the authors described carefully how they collected their sample?
4. Have the authors taken into account the number of patients who dropped out during the course of the study?
5. If the study was a trial of a treatment:
   (a) Was it randomized between two groups?

   (b) How was the randomization carried out—could it have led to bias?
   (c) Were the doctor and patient 'blind' to the treatment being given? If not, was a good reason given?
   (d) Were the treating doctor and the trial observer the same person? If so, beware.
6. If the study was of a screening technique:
   (a) Does the disorder merit screening?
   (b) Did the screening programme reach those who need it?
   (c) Was the predictive value of the test sufficient to make it a useful test (see Chapter 4)?
   (d) Is there some potential benefit for those patients identified as positive?
7. If a causal link is suggested between two factors:
   (a) Is the link consistent with the results of other studies?
   (b) Does it make biological sense?
   (c) Does the suggested 'causative' factor precede the suggested 'effect' in time?
   (d) Could the relationship be due to some other factor which has an effect on both factors in the study?
8. Were the outcome measures used clinically relevant?
9. Were there any checks on how reliably the information was recorded? Can you think of any sources of error which are not mentioned in the article?
10. Were both clinical and statistical significance considered?

HOW TO SET ABOUT ANSWERING A QUESTION!

Every project, from the simplest audit project completed by a trainee to a fully developed research project, sets out to answer a question. The principles outlined above may be applied to any size of study. The first question that the investigator must ask is 'Is the answer to the question clinically important?', and he must then decide how to answer it.

Dr Preston is interested in otitis media. He has seen articles in the journals which question the value of antibiotics in otitis media. He decided to carry out a comparison of the effect of antibiotics and placebo in patients with acute otitis media. Here were some of the questions he would have to answer when planning his trial:

1. Which patients would he include?
   —Any age?
   —Just those attending surgery?
   —How could he get his partners to include those seen on night visits?
2. Could he define otitis media? What would be the criteria for entry? He would have to get all the doctors in the study to examine some ears to see whether they could agree about the diagnosis of otitis media.

3. Would the trial be double-blind? Would the patients give consent to enter the trial? How would they be randomized, especially difficult on night or weekend calls.
4. How many patients would be needed? To calculate sample size, Dr Preston would need to know something of the natural history of otitis media from previous studies. He might well then consult a statistician on sample size calculation as well as discussing how the results would be analysed.
5. How would the results be assessed? Change in the appearance of the drum would probably be subject to substantial variation in interpretation. Would it be better to use pain, or fever, or hearing as the outcome?

CONCLUSION

The main purpose of surveys and trials is to answer questions which are of particular importance for patient care. If a result is not of clinical importance, then it will not become important however statistically significant it can be shown to be.

General practitioners who are interested in reviewing their own performance will usually be making observations on a sample of patients or of records—for example the proportion of patients with dysuria who have a positive culture of a midstream specimen of urine or the proportion of records containing a record of blood pressure. It may be appropriate to do this type of study on quite a small sample. Calculation of confidence limits as described in Chapter 4 gives an indication of how accurate an estimate made on a sample is likely to be.

Inspection of confidence limits will give an indication of the likelihood that an observed difference is due to chance or sampling error. Tests of statistical significance quantify this information and indicate just how likely it is that an observed difference is due to chance.

The performance of a statistical test is of secondary interest to observing, first, the way in which the information has been collected and, second, the actual difference which has been found. Only if the data have been collected in a valid way, and the observed differences are of clinical importance, does the test of statistical significance become relevant.

FURTHER READING

Gore, S. M. and Altman, D. G. (1982). *Statistics in practice*. British Medical Association, London.

Sackett, D. L., Haynes, R. B., Tugwell, P. (1985). *Clinical epidemiology—a basic science for clinical medicine*. Little Brown, Boston, Mass.

(Both these books have good sections on assessing clinical trials. *Statistics in practice* is designed to help the reader interpret rather than do statistics, and contains lots of examples. *Clinical epidemiology* is more detailed, and contains good sections on the interpretation of tests as well as on the interpretation of published results.)

6 What is optimal care?

Christopher Watkins

The foregoing chapters have described different ways in which the content of a doctor's work may be described and measured and have interpreted such words as 'Normality' and 'statistical significance'. In recent years a great deal has been written about the 'quality' of care provided in general practice, introducing terms like 'medical audit'. Dr Preston feels both overwhelmed and apprehensive about trying to measure quality in a task as complex as general practice. He is not alone in this.

This chapter reviews the extensive research which has been carried out in general practice over the last two decades in an attempt to come to grips with this elusive subject. While it presents an overview of the 'present state of the art', examples are included of studies which, with varying degrees of success, have made some impact on the problem. A variety of epidemiological methods have been used and perhaps Dr Preston can pick and choose from the list of references to pursue his particular area of interest.

He may find it helpful to consider the measurement of quality by first examining the structure of primary care in this country, defining what its objectives are and then considering ways in which achievements against these objectives can be measured at the practice level as well as some of the pitfalls in measuring performance.

COMPONENTS FOR A PRIMARY CARE SYSTEM

The primary system of health care in this country can be illustrated simply by the diagram presented in Fig. 6.1. The dotted line represents the borders of health care provided by professionals. The patient gains access to the system (I), then medical need is identified (II) and resolved (III) with the use of available resources. The process of medical care has an impact on outcome, and outcome in turn affects the process of care and this is denoted by the arrows in the figure. This figure provides the headings under which the quality of primary care can be examined by Dr Preston.

THE OBJECTIVES OF PRIMARY CARE

The effectiveness of any system cannot be measured unless there is a clear definition of its objectives. For the purpose of this chapter the objectives of the

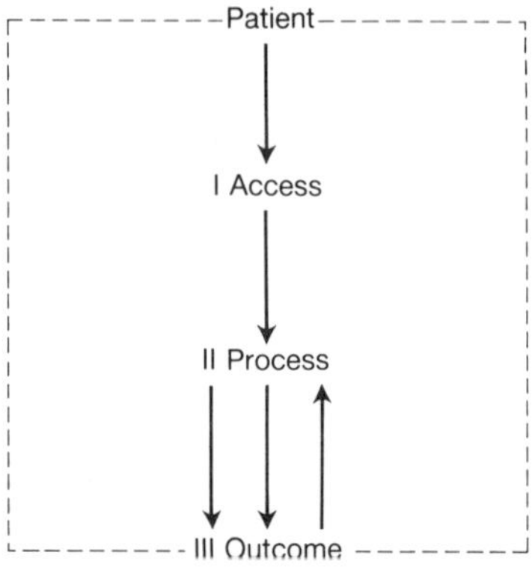

Fig. 6.1. Primary system of health care in the United Kingdom.

primary medical care system can be described as follows, and these apply whether one is examining the national objectives of the primary medical care system or the system of care provided by the individual practice:

I. Adequate access: to provide a system of medical care which is accessible and acceptable to the whole population of the country.
II. Adequacy of process: to provide a system of medical care which is capable of identifying medical need and responding appropriately.
III. Adequacy of outcome: to provide a system of medical care which can use to the maximum the available skills, manpower, and financial resources to meet the medical needs of the population.

ADEQUATE ACCESS

Access to medical care may be influenced by economic factors, e.g. the cost of care; by geographical factors, e.g. distances to be travelled and transport between the patient and the services; or by resources in terms of doctors available to provide care. In the United Kingdom none of these factors are major constraints to access. Simpler access to the primary care facilities, however, does not ensure that adequate care will be provided, since the latter may depend on the structure of the facilities which are available.

In Donabedian's (1966) classification of medical care for the purposes of quality measurement, the assessment of structure is concerned with the adequacy of facilities and equipment, medical staff qualifications, and organization. The assumption is that, without adequate structures, good processes and consequently good outcomes of care are difficult or impossible to achieve. Information collected about structure can only be interpreted in a limited way because of the many intervening variables.

A number of studies of the structure of general practice have been influential in improving standards. Perhaps the most notable of these were conducted by

Collings (1950) and Taylor (1954). These two studies pointed out the professional isolation of the single-handed general practitioner, the inadequate and inadequately equipped premises in which many general practitioners worked, and the lack of ancillary staff available to them. These and other studies led to the negotiations with the Minister of Health in 1966, which resulted in the Charter for General Practice which made it possible to modify many of these deficiencies. Another notable study of structure has been the survey of teaching practices by Irvine (1972). This survey was based on a postal questionnaire completed by 86 per cent of all 222 practices actively involved in vocational training or in undergraduate teaching or already designated for vocational training but not yet involved. Information was obtained on three axes for comparison: the medical qualification of the principals; professional, educational, and research interests of the teachers; and practice arrangements, including accommodation, arrangements of patient care, staffing, and facilities for education and research. A numerical score for the presence or absence of each item on this list was developed using a peer group of 50 doctors who were experienced teachers. The total within each axis of the activity of the practice considered enabled the performance of teaching practices of different vocational training schemes to be compared.

Simple observational studies of the content of a general practitioner's work have been influential in changing the pattern and organization of primary medical care. Examples of these are the series of studies of morbidity conducted jointly by the Royal College of General Practitioners (RCGP) and the Office of Population Censuses and Surveys, and by Morrell *et al.* in 1970, who were the first to identify the differences in content of consultations initiated by doctors, as compared with patient-initiated consultations, and who demonstrated that recording the symptoms presented in general practice as compared with diagnoses showed more clearly the diagnostic role of the doctor.

These studies have enabled the skills of a general practitioner to be defined and appropriate training programmes devised. They have also indicated ways in which the organization of primary care can be improved. For example, the introduction of appointment systems in general practice appears to have improved access by reducing waiting time (Bevan and Draper 1967) and to have improved the patients' use of the amenities provided (Stevenson 1967), and there is some evidence that it has led to a redistribution of resources in favour of the elderly and mentally ill, and to the provision of preventive services (Morrell and Kasap 1972).

It is, of course, no good having a system of primary care which is accessible if it is unacceptable to the population who make use of the service. Acceptability may be looked at in terms of the financial barriers to care, the humanity of the situation in which care is provided, and the extent to which the general practitioner lives up to the image which the population hold of him.

To a large extent patients' expectations are highly conditioned by the doctors who provide their care. The ability of doctors to change the expectations of their patients has been demonstrated by the rapid decline in the number of house calls in UK general practice. The general practitioner in this country is not so convinced of the value of the annual physical examination, which his counterpart in the USA sees as an integral part of good medical care. A comparison between the number of requests received by doctors for such examinations in each country bear witness to the ability of doctors to determine the health behaviour of their patients.

The extent to which patients are satisfied with the services provided is another and frequently measured aspect of acceptability. Cartwright's studies are particularly important in this respect as they have looked repeatedly at this important aspect of quality (Cartwright 1967; Cartwright and Anderson 1981). The general picture which has emerged from these surveys is of satisfied and appreciative patients, although in recent years there has been some criticism of the accessibility of the service. Measures of satisfaction are notoriously insensitive, however, to the doctor's clinical competence, and clearly more sensitive and specific measures are needed if these aspects of medical care are to be adequately examined.

If Dr Preston wishes to measure accessibility in his own practice, he will be concerned with the time patients wait between requesting an appointment with a doctor and the consultation. He may wish to study two aspects of this problem, i.e. the delay the patient experiences in seeing the doctor of his choice or the delay in seeing any doctor in the practice in an emergency. Equally, he may be interested in knowing the difficulties his patients experience in receiving a home visit or a call 'out-of-hours'.

There are two approaches to these issues. The first will involve him in recording requests for consultations or visits received by the receptionists and the time that elapses between the request and the consultation. The second will involve him in studying a random sample of his patients and eliciting their perception of the ease or difficulty with which a consultation or home visit may be obtained. The former has the advantage of being more objective, but the latter tells him what his patients feel, which may be more important. The former will require the co-operation of the receptionists, who will have to complete a record of the date and time of all requests for consultations and the date and time at which they are fulfilled. Dr Preston will also have to find workable ways of defining the difference between a routine as opposed to an emergency request for care. In designing such a study, he may find it helpful to refer to the work of Bevan and Draper (1967). If he adopts the latter approach, he will almost certainly have to employ a fieldworker who will conduct interviews with patients, either in their homes where the discussions will tend to be abstract or when they are attending the surgery when questions may be directed to the events surrounding the current consultation. In designing a study of this type, he will find the work of Cartwright (1967) and Cartwright and Anderson (1981) particularly helpful.

ADEQUACY OF PROCESS

The basic, if questionable, assumption made in process evaluation is that good processses of care lead to good outcome. The assessment of process is based on the relevance, completeness, or redundancy of the medical history, physical examination, laboratory investigations, diagnosis, and subsequent treatment. Many of the studies reported to have taken place as a result of the quality initiative from the RCGP have followed this pattern.

This aspect of quality measurement examines the effectiveness of the general practitioner in identifying medical need amenable to medical intervention. Two principal methods of identification exist; the first looks at the response of the general practitioner to medical demand, and the second looks at the ability to detect need which is not expressed by demand.

Response to demand

The primary diagnostic assessment in general practice operates within the context of a system providing medical care over a period of time, in which the doctor is easily accessible to the patients, where patients may be recalled for more complete evaluation if required, or be instructed to consult again if no better. The way in which the doctor responds to the presenting symptom in general practice is to attempt to detect not only a pathological process if present, but also to interpret human behaviour in response to symptoms of illness and disease. The diagnosis is made on the basis of such data as the past history of the patient, previous response to stress and disease, his social resources, and the probabilities in the primary care situation of different diseases in the presence of specific presenting symptoms, supported as necessary by physical examination and investigations.

Little is known about the procedure of problem-solving and decision-making in primary medical care, although some of these processes have been elucidated by McWhinney (1972) and Howie (1972). Hodgkin (1973) outlined a system of 'delay pattern analysis', which could be useful to the general practitioner interested in comparing his performance with those of others. Various conditions can be examined in retrospect from the time when the treatment was initiated back to the time when the patient initially perceived the symptom. His paper describes delay patterns in the diagnosis by the general practitioner for various conditions. He concluded that for the diagnosis of carcinoma of breast, rectum, and colon his performance was reasonable. For carcinoma of lung and ectopic pregnancy he felt there was room for improvement, while for myxoedema his performance left 'a great deal to be desired'. Delay patterns for referral to the specialists and waiting time to see the specialist can be analysed to throw light on the attitudes of the doctors and on the organization of the practice.

In general practice, where the doctor is often presented with conditions which are acute and self-limiting or the patient consults at a very early stage in the illness, diagnosis in terms which attribute a well-defined pathological process to the presenting condition imply a diagnostic precision which is often unjustified. This problem is discussed in more detail in Chapter 2. A more useful way of describing the clinical entities which a general practitioner encounters is to describe them in terms of symptoms and signs. One textbook of primary medical care (Cormack *et al.* 1976) has used this approach and has opened a debate with its readers as to what constitutes appropriate management for patients presenting with a given condition in general practice.

Identifying unexpressed need

The general practitioner is ideally placed to identify the 'iceberg' of treatable disease, and the potential of the primary medical care team in this respect has almost certainly not been fully realized. Ultimately the attainment of this objective must depend on population surveys. These may be undertaken at the practice level—for example, the assessment of immunization status—or by focusing on specific 'at risk' groups in the community such as the elderly or single parent families. To perform such surveys satisfactorily the general practitioner obviously needs registers which enable him to identify the target group for study with precision; ways in which these can be constructed are described in Chapter 2. Methods of measuring need are described in Chapter 3.

The setting of criteria

Before any process of care is judged to be good or bad it must be related to criteria or standards of adequate care. Most of the initial work in defining such criteria has taken place in the USA and was developed in relation to the care of the hospital in-patient. The results of this work need to be applied to UK general practice with extreme caution, although some of the methods used to devise these criteria can be employed in the UK with some modification.

In UK general practice, the quality initiative has been regarded principally as an educational exercise for those who participate in it. Sheldon (1981) has defended the use by the general practitioner of self-selected criteria for the following two reasons. First, the task of agreeing the criteria or objectives of care is itself a major part of the educational process of medical audit. It leads the doctor to review the relevant literature and to discuss the problem with other general practitioners and specialists. Second, one of the main aims of audit is to effect desired behavioural changes on the doctor where indicated, and there is increasing evidence that this change occurs only if the doctor himself plays an active part in the initial process of selecting the criteria against which his process is to be measured.

Sources of data for setting criteria

Most generally accepted clinical practices may be unrelated to patient outcomes. It is therefore important that the relevance of many of these routinely accepted practices be established in terms of patient outcomes before they become part of what is said to constitute standards of good medical care. The definition of criteria of adequacy should thus be seen as a prompt to future research rather than the enshrining of current clinical practices in immutable terms.

The sources of data used to establish criteria of medical care can be examined under two headings: non-experimental and experimental.

Non-experimental methods

Descriptive methods of study are commonly used in evaluating medical care. However, where outcomes are considered by comparative studies between practices, problems occur in interpreting the results because it is difficult to ensure that the populations being compared are indeed similar. Some data already exist which could be used to examine the quality of process of general practitioner care, but they are at present underused. The National Health Service (NHS) is already equipped to monitor and control the use and cost of prescribed drugs. For example, each prescription written in general practice is given to the patient, then deposited with the local pharmacist, who, after dispensing the prescription, forwards it to the Pricing Bureau which calculates the reimbursement. In this way prescriptions written by general practitioners can be compared with accepted norms of practice. Wade and Hood (1972) used this data source to describe the use of various drugs, including chloramphenicol, amphetamines, and bronchodilator aerosols. They demonstrated, for example, that the prescribing of chloramphenicol was confined to a few doctors, that the prescribing of amphetamines was still 'remarkably high in 1970', and that the prescribing of aerosols containing isoprenaline and adrenaline decreased only slightly over the five-year period 1966–70, despite information available to general practitioners about the dangers of such aerosols. Cochrane and Moore (1971) used the same source to show that the observed to expected consumption of vitamin B_{12} varied, according to the method of calculation, from 3:1 to 20:1.

Experimental methods

Experimental studies are directed towards determining which processes of care are best in terms of outcome. Most of these studies have used the randomized controlled design, which helps to ensure that the differences between individuals other than the method of treatment being evaluated are distributed evenly by chance between the two groups.

Using this technique, Mather *et al.* (1971) demonstrated no difference between the mortality experience of patients with myocardial infarction selected by their general practitioners for random allocation to treatment at home or in hospital. Also of interest is a randomized controlled trial which was conducted on patients presenting to general practitioners with cough and sputum (Stott and West 1976). This study showed that otherwise healthy patients who presented with cough and purulent sputum to their general practitioner did not recover more quickly when prescribed antibiotics than when on placebo treatment. Stott and West suggest that time is now ripe for another trial to test the doubtful evidence that has been used to support antibacterial treatment for most patients with purulent sputum and signs of lower respiratory infection who do not suffer from chronic bronchitis. Indeed, this experimental approach could be extended to define appropriate and inappropriate indications for the use of antibiotics in the treatment of acute infection and of psychotropic agents in the treatment of anxiety and depression in general practice. Studies like these are essential before satisfactory criteria of adequate general practitioner care are established for many of the acute conditions frequently presenting to the general practitioner.

A good example of a randomized controlled trial of management of a common condition in general practice is provided by Bain (1983). The aim of this study was to determine whether decongestants and antihistamines (a) mitigate the severity of associated symptoms of acute otitis media and upper respiratory tract infections, (b) reduce the duration of symptoms, and (c) prevent the recurrence of acute episodes during a two-month follow-up period. Cases for inclusion in the study were defined as children between the ages of three and ten with presumed acute otitis media where symptoms and signs warrant (in the doctor's judgement) the use of antibiotics. Seven practices with 22 participating general practitioners in the city of Aberdeen took part in the study during the winter months of 1980–81 and 1981–82. General practitioners were free to prescribe any antibiotic of their choice, but no additional medication. Within 24 hours of entry into the trial, a research assistant visited the homes of children to confirm that the parents understood the nature of the trial, and then issued every child and parent with 200 ml of one of the three trial drugs according to a randomized schedule. Individuals were thus assigned to treatment with pseudoephedrine, triprolidine, or a placebo. Outcome was measured from symptom diaries completed by the parents for a two-month period of time and from information about subsequent attendance to the general practitioner in the follow-up period. There was no appreciable improvement among the three treatment groups in terms of symptom relief or time taken for symptoms to resolve, nor was there any difference in the recurrence rate of acute otitis media. Side-effects were reported more often in those who received pseudoephedrine or triprolidine than in those who received placebo. The findings of this study therefore do not justify the widespread prescribing of decongestants in the management of children with acute otitis media.

The use of tracer conditions

In 1969 the Institute of Medicine of the National Academy of Sciences undertook a programme to evaluate health services received by different groups of people in the population of the USA. In developing suitable methods for assessing health status the Institute focused on the premise that specific health problems could serve as 'tracers' in analysing quality of medical care (Kessner and Kalk 1973). These tracers had to be discrete, identifiable health problems, each shedding light on how particular parts of the system work, not in isolation but in relation to one another. The basic assumption is that the way in which a doctor routinely provides care for common ailments will indicate the general quality of that care. Minimum criteria of adequate care were formulated for each tracer condition, and these criteria allowed for periodic revision. The authors of this approach to measurement of quality assume that adequate medical records are maintained, and emphasize that the results of such an exercise are only of value if they are fed back to the participating physicians.

The tracer method was used in a Canadian study of primary medical care to assess the effects of substituting nurse practitioners for physicians in primary care practice (Spitzer *et al.* 1974). In this study, known as the 'Burlington randomized trial of the nurse practitioner', patients were randomly allocated to conventional care from family physicians and to primary care for nurse practitioners. Both groups of patients had similar mortality experiences, and no differences were found in physical functional capacity, social function, or emotional function. The quality of care given to the two groups seemed similar, as assessed by a quantitative 'indicator-condition' approach. Satisfaction was high, both among patients and among professional personnel, and the new system was cost-effective. In this study the research workers departed from Kessner and Kalk's (1973) original disease-orientated or diagnostic-orientated approach to introduce presenting complaints, commonly used drugs, and the referral process for evaluation in an attempt to make this method more suitable for primary medical care.

A question which remains to be answered is the suitability of the indicator or tracer conditions selected to test the effectiveness of a doctor's special skills. Before this approach is adopted in the UK it would be worth identifying the proportion of consultations with a general practitioner which require his special skills, and indeed what these special skills are. A productive line of enquiry might be the definition of certain indicator symptoms for which criteria of adequate management could be constructed. Until indicators which require the general practitioner's particular skills have been identified there is a danger that conditions may be examined which are not true indicators of his skills, and data from which may drown those which are more sensitive.

The contribution of the medical record to studies of the process of care

In hospital practice the reputation of a doctor depends to a large extent on the opportunities that his colleagues have to observe him at work. The openness with which doctors practise in this situation is considered to be a major safeguard and has been one of the arguments used in favour of organizing general practitioners to work in groups. Ideally, the best way for an outside observer to assess a doctor's performance is to observe him at work, but it is an expensive method. Many studies have depended heavily on reviewing medical records for the adequacy of information which they contain.

Before the medical record is used extensively as a source of information about the quality of care provided, consideration needs to be given as to its validity as a data source. It cannot be inferred that the frequency of recording of variables in a medical record represents frequency of observation of the same variables. To answer this question would require a study involving an independent observer watching the doctor at work. Such studies are essential before the medical record is accepted as a valid instrument by which to measure a general practitioner's performance, but should be relatively easy to conduct using video tapes of general practitioners consulting with their patients.

Dr Preston may feel that the measurement of the process of care is too difficult and unreliable for him to initiate such studies in his practice. There are undoubtedly problems in terms of establishing criteria for high-quality care which can be accepted on a national level across a wide variety of clinical situations. There is, however, widespread agreement about the desirability of providing some preventive services, and methods of auditing this aspect of care are described in detail in Chapter 10. He may also wish to try to develop a practice policy for the management of some common conditions. He would be well advised to start by looking at acute conditions and focusing on the presenting symptoms. He might, for instance, attempt to develop a practice policy for the management of dysuria and frequency of micturition, vaginal discharge, sore throat, or sticky eyes. In doing so he will need to read the relevant literature and seek out papers which describe these problems as they present in general practice. It will be necessary for him in selecting appropriate papers to ensure that:

(1) the population studied is similar to his practice population;
(2) the symptoms were clearly defined in the study population;
(3) the process of care provided in the study population is clearly defined in terms of history-taking, examination, and investigation;
(4) the outcome justified the management described.

Having agreed a practice policy for the management of a particular presenting symptom, he will need to develop methods of recording his partners' performance. He may attempt to do this from the routine records, but, as has been indicated, this often presents problems. If he is interested in testing the validity of the new process of care which he is introducing, he may be better advised to introduce a special record card for a few months so that the partners can not only audit the care they are providing but relate this to the outcome.

ADEQUACY OF OUTCOME

Measurement of outcome can only be conducted in relation to resources allocated according to medical priorities established within the health service. Problems occur when attempting to define these priorities. For example, to what should funds be allocated? To renal dialysis units or to the provision of more district nurses? What proportion of the budget should be allocated to the hospital services and what to general medical services? A similar dilemma exists within the individual practice. How can the practice respond most effectively to public demand and yet at the same time identify unexpressed need?

Sanazaro and Williamson (1968) have described outcomes in a series of D's—death, disease, disability, discomfort, and dissatisfaction. Apart from clinical variables, outcome can be assessed in other terms, such as cost and consumer satisfaction, to provide outcome measures relevant to the condition being studied. At one end of the scale, methods have been developed which claim to measure the health of large populations and can thus be used to compare the health status of the populations of different countries. At the other end of the scale is the choice of an outcome measurement appropriate to the treatment of patients with acute infections.

The development of outcome measures for many of the acute self-limiting conditions presenting in general practice is hampered by a lack of knowledge about the natural history of such illnesses. However, some progress has been made in the long-term care of patients. A large-scale study of oral contraceptives (RCGP 1974) in general practice has revealed the ability of general practitioners to record data over a long period of time which provide useful information about the outcome of the treatment of patients with these agents. A similar study has been conducted into the outcome of abortion on subsequent physical and mental health. Another good example of a study of the natural history of illness in general practice is that conducted by Roland and Morris (1983*a*, *b*), in which the outcome of all episodes of back pain presented in general practice was described.

Particular problems exist in defining outcome in relation to the general practitioner's treatment of the chronically ill. For example, in the case of hypertension, benefits of treatment have been documented in terms of diminished mortality and morbid events such as cerebro-vascular accident (MRCWP 1985). But Sackett *et al.* (1975) showed that it is difficult to get patients to comply with treatment, even when a health education programme has taught them about their condition. One of the problems may be that hypertension is a symptomless condition. The treatment itself may produce symptoms. Bulpitt *et al.* (1974) developed a questionnaire to measure the symptoms of treated hypertensive patients, and this may be of value in the measurement of outcome of the treatment of hypertension, especially if compliance is to be obtained.

In many chronic degenerative illnesses, the potential of the general practitioner to intervene therapeutically is limited. In these situations it is important to measure outcome in terms of the level of functional impairment and the degree to which this is recognized and resources mobilized to alleviate the situation.

McDowell and Martini (1976), influenced by the work of Bergner *et al.* (1976), developed a 'socio–medical' index, examining the effect of illness on the social and psychological functioning of the patients, expressed in subjective terms. Their questionnaire has been validated and tested in different environments and the results indicate that there is good agreement between the assessments made using this questionnaire and judgements made by trained assessors. A similar questionnaire has been developed by Patrick and others and used to screen for disability in Inner London (Patrick *et al.* 1981).

The attractiveness of these and other simple indices for measuring the outcome of care is that they are easy to use and provide information about the quality of medical care cheaply. Although convenient to use, the inferences which are drawn from them are not necessarily valid. More importantly, questions may be raised about what each index means, as so many factors are involved in producing the phenomenon which the index measures. For example, if an individual or a group scores poorly on a health index, to what extent can these scores be improved by better medical care? The yardsticks against which the performance of these indices should be judged is whether patients are satisfied that the indices reflect their state of health and whether the providers of medical care are convinced that they can change the scores on these indices by better medical treatment.

Setting standards

Under the present arrangement in the NHS the individual general practitioner agrees to provide continuous care at all times for the patients on his list. He also agrees to make available to his patients, as required, specialist, nursing, and social services. Beyond these broad commitments he is not required to justify the appropriateness of his clinical judgements. In maternity care, however, the general practitioner has to satisfy local obstetric committees of his competence to practice obstetrics before he is paid on the highest scale for this work.

Yet there are signs that the clinical competence of general practitioners will be exposed to greater scrutiny in the future. Of interest in this respect is the wording on form FP1001 provided by the Family Practitioners Committee, used by the general practitioner to claim a fee for providing contraceptive services for his patient. This states that the doctor will provide contraceptive services 'having regard to and being guided by modern authoritative medical opinion, such as the advice given in the *Handbook of contraceptive practice* issued by the Standing Medical Advisory Committee' (DHSS, Scottish Home and Health Dept., Welsh Office, 1979). Such a statement, signed by the general practitioner, implies that the clinical care that he provides may be examined to see that it reaches an adequate standard. This appears to be the first time that the standards of clinical care provided by UK general practitioners have been laid open to such scrutiny. This development implies that the standards of general practitioner care for other conditions may be examined in the future. Who is to set these standards of clinical care, and how are these standards to be developed? Before the quality of medical care can be said to be good or bad, there must be some agreement on what should be done for the patients.

Once the diagnosis has been made, management of acute surgical problems would appear to be easy. However, Dudley (1974) found that it took no less than 18 attempts before agreement could be reached by surgeons in his London teaching hospital on how patients presenting with massive upper gastro-intestinal haemorrhage should be managed. How much more difficult it is for the general practitioner to define standards of care, when it is difficult to make even a precise diagnosis in a high proportion of patients. For example, in a study of symptom interpretation in general practice, Morrell (1971) found that for symptoms referable to the skin and respiratory tract, precise diagnoses were recorded at between 60 and 90 per cent of the consultations. However, for the symptoms of abdominal pain and gastro-intestinal disturbance, the 'presumptive' level of diagnosis was recorded at less than 30 per cent of consultations.

The general practitioner frames his diagnoses in physical, social, and psychological terms. Because of the complexities of this diagnostic process, Acheson (1975) suggested that general practitioners should take the initiative in developing methods of measuring the quality of care that they provide. He proposed that they should concentrate on simple physical problems, for which it should be relatively straightforward to develop standards of care, rather than try to measure the quality of care provided for patients suffering from problems with a high social or psychological content.

A good recent example of audit of medical care is that conducted by Saunders *et al.* (1986). The purposes of this study were to assess what proportion of these patients presenting to their general practitioners with dyspepsia had evidence of underlying disease and to investigate in a randomized controlled trial the effectiveness of the treatment of dyspepsia with ranitidine. Guidelines could then be provided for general practitioners on the management of dyspepsia in general practice. All patients aged 18–65 years presenting to the participating general practitioners with epigastric or retrosternal pain or discomfort related to meals of at least two weeks' duration were recruited. Endoscopic examination was performed on each patient on entry to the study and then each individual whose symptoms persisted for six to eight weeks was assigned at random to treatment with ranitidine or to a placebo. Symptom diaries were maintained by patients to measure outcome, and information was extracted from the medical records of the participants about treatment prescribed for dyspepsia over the year following entry to the study. Thirty per cent of patients recruited had no endoscopic abnormality and, of the remainder, one-third had two or more lesions. Three patients had malignancies. All of these were over the age of 50. There was no characteristic history or pattern of distribution that could be accurately related to underlying disease. Complete remission of symptoms occurred in 76 per cent of patients who were taking ranitidine and in 55 per cent of those who were taking placebo. Of those with non-ulcer dyspepsia, significantly more became symptom-free taking ranitidine compared with placebo.*

As a result of this study, the following guidelines were suggested by the authors of the paper to family doctors:

> Treat patients with dyspepsia without investigation if it is their first episode; if they relapse, arrange for endoscopy and other tests as appropriate; those over the age of 40 may have a malignancy and it may be prudent to investigate them at the outset (Saunders *et al.* 1986, p. 668).

In general practice the contrast between setting standards of care for patients with acute and those with chronic disease is marked. Once the diagnosis of chronic disease is made, the standards of clinical care which are set should ideally be based on the results of studies which relate the process of care to outcome or, alternatively, on what is generally accepted by most general practitioners as 'good practice'. Relatively few studies have related changes in process to outcome of care for chronic disease. Major difficulties in such studies are that the alteration of medical management has to be sustained over a considerable length of time, and large numbers of patients have to be studied before an appreciable change in outcome can be observed.

It is difficult to rely on what general practitioners accept as 'good' or 'adequate' clinical practice and to establish standards against which the performance of other general practitioners may be judged. Watkins (unpublished thesis, 1980) showed that a group of eight general practitioners could not reach agreement on what formed minimal essential criteria of clinical care of patients suffering from diabetes or cardiac failure. In their discussions the group recognized the problems of taking into account the social and psychological aspects of care of patients with chronic disease and attempted to restrict their discussions purely to the physical aspect of care. However, the way in which the doctors perceived the psychological and social circumstances of the individual patient were felt by the group to be an important factor in determining how frequently observations were made.

Another problem in attempting to set standards for the clinical care of patients with chronic disease is that many of these diseases are due to degeneration of organs or systems in the body, for which there is no specific treatment available. The frequency with which clinical observations are made

*The controlled trial demonstrated the treatment of dyspepsia with ranitidine was both effective and safe.

by a doctor may be irrelevant as the doctor cannot intervene to alter the progress of the disease. For example, the treatment of a patient with chronic bronchitis or osteoarthritis can only be directed towards the alleviation of symptoms and disability. Faced with a patient with chronic incurable disease, the ability of the general practitioner to make diagnoses of its social and psychological effects, and to treat these, may be of greater importance than his ability to manage the physical aspects of the disease.

Having read this chapter, Dr Preston may feel that any attempt to alter the management of illness in his practice and relate this to the outcome of the care provided is likely to fail. This would be a very defeatest attitude. In the management of prevention and in the management of acute illness there is often good evidence to show that the process of care does in fact influence the outcome and that experiments in these fields would be rewarding. In the case of chronic disease the problems are more difficult, but this is what research is all about. The development of well-validated methods of measuring health and disability has opened up opportunities for measuring outcome in the management of chronic disease. The provision of conventional medical care may not influence outcome in terms of conventional medical measurements of disease. The introduction of, for instance, physiotherapy, occupational therapy, and social services may markedly influence, however, the health status of individuals suffering from chronic degenerative diseases. By carrying out such studies he would advance knowledge of the management of chronic disease in general practice and contribute to the discussion about optimal care.

REFERENCES

Acheson, H. W. K. (1975). Medical audit and general practice. *Lancet* **1,** 511–13.

Bain, D. J. G. (1983). Can the clinical course of acute otitis media be modified by systemic decongestant or antihistamine treatment? *British Medical Journal* **287,** 654–6.

Bergner, M., *et al.* (1976). The sickness impact profile: conceptual formulation and methodology for the development of a health status measure. *International Journal of Health Services* **6,** 393–415.

Bevan, J. M. and Draper, G. J. (1967). *Appointment systems in general practice.* Oxford University Press.

Bulpitt, C. J., Dollery, C. T., and Carne, S. (1974). A symptom questionnaire for hypertensive patients. *Journal of Chronic Diseases* **27,** 309–23.

Cartwright, A. (1967). *Patients and their doctors.* Routledge and Kegan Paul, Andover, Hants.

Cartwright, A. and Anderson, R. (1981). *General practice revisited: a second study of patients and their doctors.* Tavistock Publications, Andover, Hants.

Cochrane, A. L. and Moore, F. (1971). Expected and observed values for the prescription of Vitamin B_{12} in England and Wales. *British Journal of Preventive and Social Medicine* **25,** 147–51.

Collings, J. S. (1950). General practice in England today. *Lancet* **1,** 555–85.

Cormack. J., Morrell, D. C., and Marinker, M. (1987). *Practice*. Kluwer, London.

DHSS (Department of Health and Social Security), Scottish Home and Health Department, Welsh Office (1978). *Handbook of contraceptive practice*, Standing Medical Advisory Committee of the Central Health Services Council, The Secretary of State for Social Services, and The Secretary of State for Wales.

Donabedian, A. (1966). Evaluating the quality of medical care. *Milbank Memorial Fund Quarterly*, **44,** (No. 3, part 2), 166–206.

Dudley, H. (1974). Necessity for surgical audit. *British Medical Journal* **1,** 275–7.

Hodgkin, G. K. (1973). Evaluating the doctor's work. *Journal of the Royal College of General Practitioners* **23,** 759–67.

Howie, J. G. R. (1972). Diagnosis—the Achilles heel? *Journal of the Royal College of General Practitioners* **22,** 310–15.

Irvine, D. (1972). *Teaching practices. Reports from General Practice 15*. Royal College of General Practitioners, London.

Kessner, D. M. and Kalk, C. E. (1973). *A strategy for evaluating health services. Conclusions: recommendation and summary. Contrasts in health status, Vol. 2.* Institute of Medicine, National Academy of Sciences, Washington DC.

McDowell, I. and Martini, C. (1976). Problems and new directions in the evaluation of primary care. *International Journal of Epidemiology* **5,** 247–50.

McWhinney, I. R. (1972). Problem-solving and decision making in primary medical practice. *Proceedings of the Royal Society of Medicine* **65,** 934–8.

Mather, H. G., *et al.* (1971). Acute myocardial infarction: home and hospital treatment. *British Medical Journal* **3,** 334–8.

Morrell, D. C. and Kasap, H. S. (1972). The effect of an appointment system on demand for medical care. *International Journal of Epidemiology* **1,** 143–51.

Morrell, D. C., Gage, H. G., and Robinson, N. A. (1970). Patterns of demand in general practice. *Journal of the Royal College of General Practitioners* **19,** 331–42.

Morrell, D. C., Gage, H. G., and Robinson, N. A. (1971). Symptoms in general practice. *Journal of the Royal College of General Practitioners* **21,** 32–43.

MRCWP (Medical Research Council Working Party) (1985). MRC trial of treatment for mild hypertension. *British Medical Journal* **104,** 291–297.

Patrick, D. L., Darby, S. C., Green, S., Horton, G., Locker, D., and Wiggins, R. D. (1981). Screening for disability in the inner city. *Journal of Epidemiology and Community Health* **35,** 65–70.

RCGP (Royal College of General Practitioners) (1974). *Oral contraceptives and health.* Pitman, London.

Roland, M. O., and Morris, R. W. (1983*a*). A study of the natural history of back paid—part I: development of a reliable and sensitive measure of disability in low back pain. *Spine* **8,** 141–4.

Roland, M. O. and Morris, R. W. (1983*b*). A study of the natural history of back pain—part II: development of guidelines for trials of treatment in primary care. *Spine* **8,** 145–50.

Sackett, D. L., *et al.* (1975). Randomised clinical trial of strategies for improving medication compliance in primary hypertension. *Lancet* **1,** 1205–7.

Sanazaro, P. J. and Williamson, J. W. (1968). End results of patient care: a provisional classification based on reports by internists. *Medical Care* **6,** 123–30.

Saunders, J. H. B., Oliver, R. J., and Higson, D. L. (1986). Dyspepsia: incidence of non-ulcer disease in a controlled trial of ranitidine in general practice. *British Medical Journal* **292,** 665–8.

Sheldon, M. G. (1981). Medical audit in general practice. *Journal of the Royal College of General Practitioners*, Occasional Paper 20.

Spitzer, W. O., *et al.* (1974). The Burlington randomised trial of the nurse practitioners. *New England Journal of Medicine* **290**, 251–6.

Stevenson, J. S. K. (1967). Appointment systems in general practice: how patients use them. *British Medical Journal* **2**, 827–9.

Stott, N. C. H. and West, R. R. (1976). Randomised controlled trial of antibiotics in patients with cough and purulent sputum. *British Medical Journal* **2**, 556–9.

Taylor, S. (1954). *Good general practice*. Oxford University Press.

Wade, O. L. and Hood, H. (1972). Prescribing of drugs reported to cause adverse reactions. *British Journal of Preventive Social Medicine* **26**, 205–11.

Watkins, C. J. (1980). Experimental research into the quality of medical care delivered to patients suffering from chronic disease. Unpublished Ph.D thesis, University of London.

7 Are psycho-social factors measurable?

Leone Ridsdale

In Chapter 3 the terms health, disease, illness, and sickness were discussed in the context of measuring the needs for medical care in the population. One of the problems which concerns Dr Preston is the tenuous relationship between disease and demands for medical care. This chapter is concerned with considering some of the factors which influence patients in their decision to seek medical care. Many of these are psycho-social influences which may have an impact on the consulting behaviour of patients suffering from such different problems as streptococcal sore throats and depression. This chapter describes how stress, life events, and social ties may be measured and how they relate to disease, illness, and sickness. Some of the methods described may be used by general practitioners who wish to answer questions about their own practices. Others are more suited to in-depth epidemiological studies of the aetiology of disease and illness behaviour.

SOCIAL CHARACTERISTICS

If Dr Preston wishes to have a greater understanding of the factors which influence the demand for his services, he must begin to identify and record information about the social characteristics which affect consulting behaviour. Characteristics such as age and sex have been described in Chapter 2. This chapter is concerned with social and psychological characteristics.

Marital status is not routinely recorded. The general practitioner requiring information about this may either have to conduct a survey of the particular patients he is studying or persuade his partners to record this information routinely. Ethnic differences also determine behaviour and particularly beliefs. Very little information about ethnicity has been routinely recorded in general practice.

Important variations in health and consulting behaviour are associated with differences in social class. This is not routinely recorded in general practice. Classification of this kind presents considerable theoretical and practical problems. Class is not something that exists like a broken leg! A variety of factors may be taken into consideration in constructing a socio–economic classification, such as income, type of housing, education, and occupation. To a certain extent the selection of one factor as an indicator of class is arbitrary. But, historically, occupation has been selected as the principal indicator of social class. Since 1911 the Registrar General's classification of occupations has been the commonest instrument used. The broad categories and the percentage of men so classified are as follows (OPCS Registrar General, Scotland 1984):

(I) professional (for example, doctor, lawyer) (5 per cent);
(II) intermediate (for example, nurse, schoolteacher) (19 per cent);
(III) skilled non-manual (for example, secretary, shop assistant) (13 per cent) (N);
(III) skilled manual (for example, butcher, carpenter) (37 per cent) (M);
(IV) partly skilled (for example, postman) (17 per cent);
(V) unskilled (for example, cleaner, labourer) (8 per cent).

The advantage of using a nationally accepted classification in research is that it gives the investigator the opportunity to compare his results with the results of other studies. But this classification does have limitations. It came into being at a time when women contributed little to the family income, and divorce was relatively uncommon. Single women are generally categorized according to their own occupation and married women according to their husbands' occupation. Separated and divorced women and retired people are difficult to classify. The general practitioner who tries to classify the women and children who present to him will often find it difficult to obtain this precise occupational information.

These practical and conceptual limitations have led researchers to develop new methods of classification. General practitioners intuitively classify their patients' socio–economic status by looking at the address on the records. 'A classification of residential neighbourhoods', the ACORN code (Anon 1983), was developed for marketing purposes to identify areas with different patterns of consumer behaviour. It groups people according to the type of residential area in which they live. With the use of census data, residential areas can be related to other social variables such as age structure, employment, housing, and family structure. The practical advantage of this system is that each individual can be classified simply by his postal code. Morgan and Chinn (1983) have shown that ACORN is as good as the Registrar General's classification at explaining variations in health and service use and at identifying high-risk groups. The information is much easier to obtain because it depends simply on knowing the postcode. Access to the ACORN code, however, may be costly unless the district health authority or region has purchased this information and is prepared to make it available to interested professionals such as general practitioners.

Social characteristics and consulting behaviour

Morbidity statistics from general practice (RCGP, OPCS, and DHSS 1982, 1986; Crombie 1984) demonstrate that young children and the elderly consult more than those intermediate in age. Women of child-bearing age consult more than their male counterparts. Single men and women consult less often than their married contemporaries. Patient-initiated consultations vary little by social class, and patients in the lower social classes attend less frequently for preventive procedures (see Fig. 7.1).

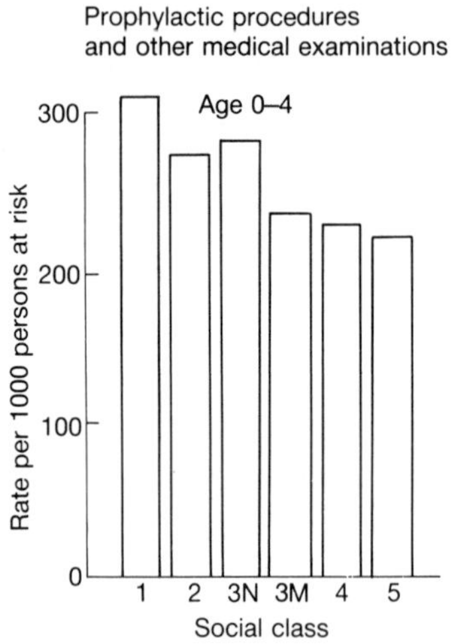

Fig. 7.1. Patient consulting rates per person at risk by social class for preventive, prophylactic, and immunization procedures. [From RCGP, OPCS, and DHSS (1982, p. 17).]

This information poses more questions than it answers. It is clear that disease or risk of disease is not necessarily related to consulting behaviour. Women live longer but consult more often when they are of child-bearing age. Married men and women have lower mortality than the single but consult more frequently. People in lower social classes have a higher risk of disease but initiate consultations at the same rate as those of higher occupational groups. Lower occupational groups make less use of preventive services provided by general practitioners.

Several questions arise. What other factors can be associated with disease and consulting behaviour? How do psychological factors affect disease and consulting behaviour? Why do women of child-bearing age consult more? How is consulting behaviour related to a patient's social role in the community?

Psychological factors and physical disease

Why do certain patients develop illness while others remain healthy? Common infections are endemic in the community, but patients vary in their resistance or vulnerability to them. Individual vulnerability to infection may be increased by psychological stress. How can a hypothesis such as this be tested in general practice?

Meyer and Haggerty (1962) selected 16 families of similar socio–economic status, all of whom had two or more children. For one year they cultured the throats of all family members every three weeks for group A beta-haemolytic streptococcus. Every four months they measured antistreptolysin O titres in the blood. They conducted serial interviews with the families and asked them to keep a diary of illness, therapy, and life events.

They found that 21 per cent of the throat cultures were positive for beta-haemolytic streptococci. However, only 47 per cent of those with positive cultures developed any illness. They then examined the record of acute family stress two weeks before and two weeks after acquisition of illness. They found that streptococcal acquisition and illness was four times as likely to be preceded by as to be followed by acute stress. They also found that chronic stress was important. After an acquisition of streptococci, antistreptolysin O increases were seen in only 21 per cent of the patients in the low-stress families, compared to 49 per cent of those patients in moderate–high stress families.

This prospective study suggests a chain of causality. If person A experiences psychological stress, this increases his vulnerability to an infectious agent which will then be more likely to cause disease (see Fig. 7.2). However, if someone is exposed to noxious influences like stress and infectious agents separately or, like person B, in reverse order, they will be less likely to precipitate illness. The additive effect depends on the order in which an individual is exposed to noxious influences.

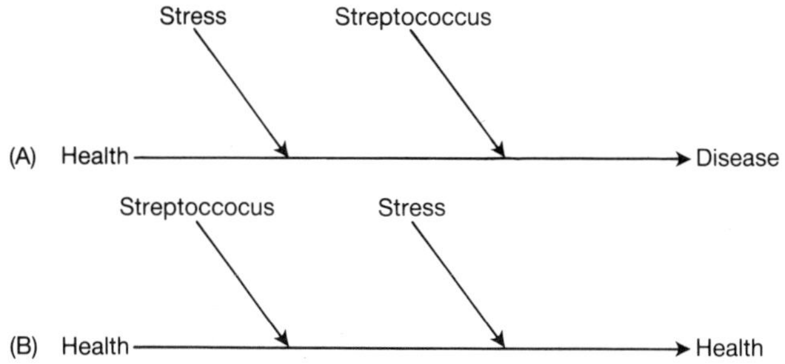

Fig. 7.2. Effect of noxious influences: (A) synergistic; (B) simple.

The chronology of events is of critical importance if the purpose of general practice research is to tease out causal relationships. Cross-sectional studies, as described in Chapter 3, yield a picture like a still-life photograph of a process which is evolving over time. But the general practitioner sees a continuous process of events and responses over time. The chain of causality is elucidated more clearly in a prospective study in which events and responses are documented when they happen, as in a moving film. To a greater extent, Meyer and Haggerty (1962) achieved this. But even prospective studies generally contain some retrospective element. They also involve more planning and time. These issues will be taken up in the next example.

Social factors and psychological disease

Although the life-expectancy of females is longer than their male counterparts, general practice morbidity surveys show that women of child-bearing age consult more. Sixty per cent of general practice consultations are with female patients. Part of this seeming excess can be simply explained. Women have a complex reproductive role. A proportion of their visits are for family planning, perinatal, and gynaecological care. But women also visit their doctors twice as often with problems that are diagnosed as psychological. Depression, in particular, is diagnosed twice as often in women. An organic predisposition cannot be excluded. However, the phenomenon has stimulated research into the social causes of psychological disease.

Brown and Harris (1978) postulated that most clinical depression is an understandable response to adversity. They proposed a model in which life events and difficulties act as provoking agents in the genesis of depressive disorder. To test this hypothesis they undertook a cross-sectional study of women in Camberwell, London.

Brown and Harris (1978) noted that disease may be unrelated to visits to the doctor. They therefore decided to pick a random sample of women in the community as well as women who were already receiving medical care. Previous research had demonstrated an association between life events and psychiatric disease. Hitherto, however, the research instruments used were criticized for potential bias. Self-report questionnaires had been used which would allow respondents to give priority to past life events in the light of their current emotional state.

The Camberwell study was investigator-based. Interviewers were trained at the Institute of Psychiatry to use a standardized interview called the Present State Examination (PSE). The PSE is based on a glossary of psychotic and neurotic symptoms (Wing *et al.* 1981). Semi-structured interviews were undertaken and the interviewer enquired about life events and difficulties in the year prior to interview. A panel of experienced raters made consensus judgements about the likely meaning and expected stressfulness of events and difficulties. This rating was made with information about the particular biography and circumstances of the person, but ignoring what she said about her reaction.

In Fig. 7.3 the percentage of women with depression in Camberwell who were identified as cases or borderline cases in the three months before interview is related to their marital status, social class, and children's age. Women who developed depression were much more likely to have experienced severe events or major difficulties prior to its onset than women without depression. However, only one in five women experiencing a provoking agent went on to develop depression. Brown and Harris (1978) demonstrated that women who developed depression experienced more vulnerability factors. Vulnerability factors do not cause depression on their own but lower the individual's threshold, increasing the risk of depression when a provoking agent occurs. Vulnerability factors included the loss of mother before 11 years of age, three or more children under the age of 14, and lack of employment outside the home.

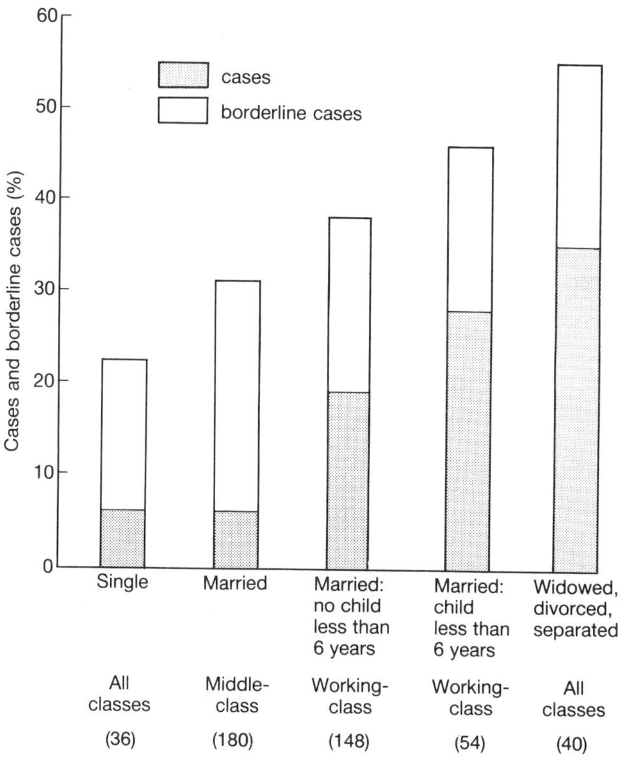

Fig. 7.3. Percentage of women identified as suffering from depression in relation to civil status and social class in the Camberwell study.

However, the key vulnerability factor concerned an assessment of the women's relationship in terms of intimacy and ability to confide in their husbands, boy-friends, or women friends. In the face of a severe event or major difficulty, those who were rated lower in terms of the quality of a confiding relationship were more likely to develop depression.

To further unravel the temporal relationships involved in the aetiology of depression, Brown *et al.* (1986) undertook a prospective study of mothers in Islington, London. Working-class women with a child living at home were selected since previous research suggested that they were particularly likely to develop a depressive disorder. The investigation was conducted in two phases, approximately one year apart. At first contact, measures of the quality of personal ties were collected. In the second phase measures were made of life events, stress, and social support received during any crisis in the intervening year. At both points of contact details were obtained of any psychiatric disorder in the preceding year.

In this two-stage study, the investigators were able to assess the support given by 'core ties' before and after stresses had occurred. A core tie was defined as a husband, lover, or someone named as very close at first contact. Single mothers mostly named other women as close ties, about half of whom were kin, mostly mothers or sisters.

The research confirmed previous findings that the majority of instances of depression follow events with long-term threat or major difficulties lasting two years or more. Brown *et al.* (1986) tested the hypothesis that confiding in a 'core tie' at first interview would protect against depression if a crisis occurred. However, they found this only to hold where the expected support in a crisis (based on information collected at the first interview with the woman) was actually forthcoming in any crisis in the follow-up year. If this confirmation of support occurred there was a very much reduced risk of the woman developing clinical depression.

The investigators found that, in the case of married women who were receiving support at the time of first contact, 40 per cent did not receive support at the time of a crisis in the follow-up year. The women 'let down' in this way had a particularly high rate of depression. In contrast, confiding in core ties by single mothers was very highly related to later crisis support and to a lower risk of depression. However, single mothers were a good deal more likely to experience events with long-term threat or major difficulties.

The time order of stress, support, and psychiatric disorder is crucial. This study illustrates how a sophisticated two-stage method can be used to investigate the complex relationship between social phenomena and disease in the community.

Symptoms and consulting behaviour

Meyer and Haggerty (1962) showed the relationship between stress and organic disease. Brown and Harris (1978) and Brown *et al.* (1986) showed the relationship between social factors and psychological disease. The latter deliberately studied women in the community separately from their demand for medical care, but Dr Preston is also concerned about the frequency of his consultations with women of child-bearing age.

Morrell and Wale (1976) and Banks *et al.* (1975) made a detailed study of 198 women aged 20–44 years who were registered with one practice. The women were asked to complete a health diary for a period of four weeks during the study year. A general practitioner record card was inserted into their medical records to provide objective measures of the medical care delivered. Information on who initiated the consultations and details of symptoms and diagnosis were recorded for one year.

They found that 54 per cent of consultations were initiated by doctors and 46 per cent by the women themselves. A subgroup of 24 per cent of women did not consult the doctor at all during the study year. The mean frequency of actual patient-initiated consultations was 2.18 per person.

In analysing the diaries, an episode of symptoms was defined to be a group of consecutive days on which the same symptom was recorded. The mean number of episodes of symptoms per diary was 6.2, with an average duration of 1.6 days. Extrapolating from the diary experience, the investigators estimated that the women experienced 81 espisodes of symptoms per year, so that for every 37 symptom episodes experienced by patients, there was one patient-initiated consultation.

The researchers were able to relate the types of symptoms experienced to those which were presented at consultations (Fig. 7.4). Clearly there is a difference between the type of symptoms experienced and those presented to the doctor. One episode of headache in 184 leads a patient to consult, but one in 18 episodes of sore throat leads to a consultation. This suggests that symptoms are evaluated differently in terms of significance. The researchers also demonstrated that individuals with higher scores on objective measures of anxiety were more likely both to record and to present symptoms to the doctors.

Unemployment and consultating behaviour

The studies which have been described have focused on the social and psychological factors which influence illness and consulting behaviour in women. Some life events such as unemployment have a major effect on men, and general practitioners may wish to study the effects of these events on illness and consultations.

Beale and Nethercote (1986*a*, *b*) undertook a longitudinal study in general practice of patients who were made redundant by factory closure. This was a case-control study, so the patients were compared to others who were fully employed during the study period. Consultations, episodes of illness, and referrals to and attendances at hospital out-patient departments were

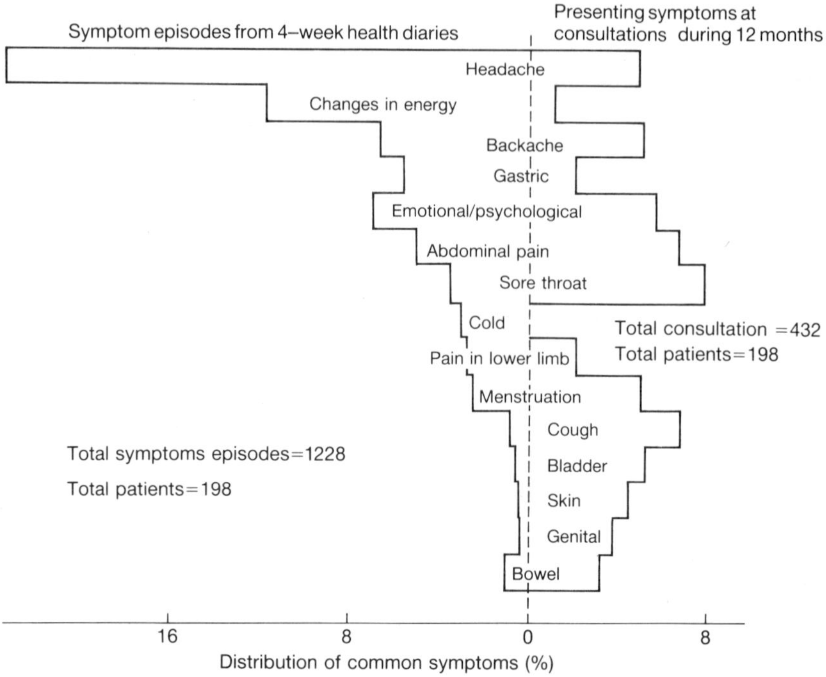

Fig. 7.4. Relationship between episodes of symptoms recorded in health diaries and symptoms presented at consultations.

monitored. The longitudinal study covered eight years. During the first four years, jobs were secure among the study group. During the next two years they were threatened with job loss, and the final two years followed redundancy.

Beale and Nethercote found that in the study group older patients with a previously low consulting rate showed a 150 per cent increase in the number of consultations, and a 70 per cent increase in the number of episodes of illness when compared with controls. Among these patients there was also a 160 per cent increase in the number of referrals to hospital out-patient departments, and a 200 per cent increase in the number of attendances at out-patient departments. These changes were found to occur two years before actual job loss, when the workers learned that their jobs were in jeopardy. The threat of unemployment was associated with increased consultations among male and female workers and this association increased with age. However, men and women in the five years before expected retirement responded differently. In this age group there was a significant increase in consultations among male employees but not among female employees.

This study measured the relationship between threat of redundancy and consulting behaviour in one community. It exemplifies the potential of general practice research in documenting the relationship between social factors and consulting behaviour.

Concepts and measures

There appears to be a mismatch between the needs for care and service use. Some patients demand consultations for what appear to be trivial complaints, others underutilize the service despite quite evident sickness. In addition, many practitioners are confused by widely differing figures about the iceberg of disease and the inference drawn in the Black Report (1980; see also Townsend and Davidson 1982) that medical care is distributed unfairly. Differing reports about morbidity beg two questions:

(1) What is sickness?
(2) How is it measured?

Dr Preston may widen his frame of reference by considering the effect of psycho-social pressures in the community. In doing so he will find several instruments which he can use to measure sickness in the practice population. These include:

(1) diaries;
(2) standardized interviews;
(3) general practitioner record cards.

Each of these instruments can be used to collect data. Information can be accumulated and analysed. The results can then be used to make inferences about sickness in the community. Some of the different results and inferences which followed the Black Report (1980) stemmed from issues of measurement. Different surveys gave priority to different indicators, and data was analysed in different ways.

More fundamental is the problem of definition. What is sickness? Different concepts have been described. There is no generally agreed definition. The concept shifts over time and is related to services available and used. If researchers operationalize definitions in different ways, their results may seem incongruous. For example, Cartwright (1967) found that one-quarter of the 420 general practitioners she surveyed felt that more than 50 per cent of surgery consultations were for trivial complaints. In contrast to this, Hannay (1979) found that less than 10 per cent of patients reported taking trivial medical conditions to their general practitioner. These results seem incongruous. How can the different figures be explained? The surveys were done at different times and in different places. Ten per cent of patients may consult frequently and account for the 50% consultations for trivial complaints. But the most likely reason for the different figures is that the researchers were asking questions which tapped the perceptions of different groups of people. Doctors and patients will tend to have different definitions of trivia. Similarly they tend to define sickness differently. The same word has overlapping but different meanings for different social groups. When research is undertaken in a social context, a major challenge is to define concepts and to recognize how shifts of meaning can lead to incongruity and confusion.

REFERENCES

Anon (1983). *ACORN— users guide.* Market Analysis Division, 59–62 High Holborn, London WC1V 6DX.

Banks, M. H., Beresford, S. A. A., Morell, D. C., Waller, J. J., and Watkins, C. J. (1975). Factors influencing demand for primary medical care in women aged 20–44 years: a preliminary report. *International Journal of Epidemiology* **4,** 189–95.

Beale, N. and Nethercott, S. (1986*a*). Job-loss and health—the influence of age and previous morbidity. *Journal of the Royal College of General Practitioners* **36,** 261–4.

Beale, N. and Nethercott, S. (1986*b*). Job-loss and morbidity in a group of employees nearing retirement age. *Journal of the Royal College of General Practitioners* **36,** 265–6.

Brown, G. W. and Harris, T. O. (1978). *Social origins of depression.* Tavistock Publications, Andover, Hants.

Brown, G. W., Andrews, B., Harris, T., Adler, Z., and Bridge, L. (1986). Social support, self-esteem and depression. *Psychological medicine* **16(4),** 813–31.

Cartwright, A. (1967). *Patients and their doctors.* Routledge and Kegan Paul, Andover, Hants.

Crombie, D. L. (1984). *Social class and health status inequality or difference.* Occasional Paper 25, Royal College of General Practitioners, London.

Department of Health and Social Security, London. *Inequalities in health.* Report of a Research Working Group chaired by Sir Douglas Black (1980).

Hannay, D. R. (1979). The symptom iceberg. Routledge and Kegan Paul, Andover, Hants.

Meyer, J. N. and Haggerty, R. J. (1962). Streptococcol infections in families. *Pediatrics* **29, 539–49.**

Morgan, M. and Chinn, S. (1983). ACORN group, social class and child health. *Journal of Epidemiology and Community Health* **37**(3), 196–203.

Morrell, D. C. and Wale, C. J. (1976). Symptoms perceived and recorded by patients. *Journal of the Royal College of General Practitioners* **26,** 398–403.

OPCS (Office of Population Censuses and Surveys) Registrar General, Scotland (1984). *Census 1981. Economic Activity Great Britain.* HMSO, London.

RCGP, OPCS, and DHSS (Royal College of General Practitioners, Office of Popultion Censuses and Surveys, and Department of Health and Social Security) (1982). *Morbidity statistics from general practice. Socio-economic analysis.* Studies on Medical and Population Subjects, No. 46. HMSO, London.

RCGP, OPCS, and DHSS (Royal College of General Practitioners, Office of Population Censuses and Surveys, and Department of Health and Social Security) (1986). *Morbidity statistics from general practice. Third National Study, 1981–82.* HMSO, London.

Townsend, P. and Davidson, N. (1982). *Inequalities in health.* Penguin Books, Harmondsworth, Middx.

Wing, J. K., Bebbington, P., and Robins, L. N. (1981). *What is a case?—The problem of definition in psychiatric community surveys.* Grant McIntyre, London.

8 What do my patients think?

Leone Ridsdale

In considering his patients' problems, Dr Preston wonders how their understanding of illness and their health beliefs differ from his own. Populations can be subdivided according to common characteristics like age, sex, marital status, and social class. In Chapter 7 it was shown that these common characteristics are associated with different risks of disease and patterns of consulting behaviour.

The general practitioner finds himself stationed at the crossroads between the community and hospital care. His concept of sickness or trivia have overlapping but different meanings from those of his patients. When a young principal finds his ideas and expectations at odds with his experience, he will ask: What do my patients think?

This question can be posed in an anthropological or sociological way. Patients can be considered as social groups who try to explain their experience meaningfully and evolve theories about symptoms, causes of disease, and remedies. Some of the variations in patients' ideas and consulting behaviour can be related to group characteristics, like age, gender, ethnicity, and class. But as people vary individually, some differences cannot be explained as group phenomena.

PATIENTS' BELIEFS

What methods are available to obtain information about patients' health beliefs?

Most epidemiological research aims to define the question and the classes of information sought early in the study. The researcher creates clear operational definitions of the units and qualities he will measure. He anticipates how he will classify variables, so that they can be quantified in a pre-arranged numerical way.

The researcher approaching health beliefs may take a different approach. First, the units and qualities may not be known or they cannot be so readily defined at the outset of the research programme. Some of the characteristics of the population may only emerge in the process of the study.

Community surveys often collect information through structured questionnaires. Structured questionnaires may be sent to patients or given to them at the surgery. The same words are used in questioning all respondents and these questions are posed in the same order. This is an appropriate method of data gathering when factual information is required. However, it may be less suitable when information is sought concerning beliefs about sensitive issues like symptoms, their cause, and possible remedies. Ideas like this are not often publicly expressed and direct questions may evoke stereotyped answers.

Information about lay beliefs is therefore better obtained by interviewing people in the community. Usually a semi-structured interview is undertaken. The interviewer formulates questions in the words that seem most appropriate for each respondent and varies the sequence of questions responsively. Interviewers seek the classes of information needed in a flexible way. This is analagous to the technique of an experienced doctor taking a medical history, but the doctor is generally looking for different types of information.

A third method of interviewing may be used when issues are not so clearly defined that they can be specified in advance. This is the case in the pilot phase of a study which is opening up a new field of research. The method is an unstructured interview and takes the form of a prolonged conversation. The method permits exploration and the development of ideas. It is more akin to the technique used by a general practitioner when he is not sure what the problem is. The open-ended approach permits the characteristics of the responses to emerge. These last two methods are time-consuming and they require trained interviewers, so the number of people interviewed tends to be small.

As the characteristics of the responses emerge, the researcher can generate a systems of classification. For example, some respondents may be found more often to attribute the cause of disease to germs; others may be found more often to attribute the cause of disease to stress. These two explanations can form the basis of a conceptual classification. The first part of a survey such as this tends to be descriptive. The researcher may generate hypotheses during the collection and analysis of his data.

Lay beliefs about infection

During his morning surgery, Dr Preston saw more patients with infection than anything else. Most of the infections affected the respiratory tract. He wonders if people are consulting more frequently with respiratory infections. The third general practice morbidity survey (RCGP, OPCS, and DHSS 1986) shows that consultation frequency is rising for upper respiratory infections, but falling for influenza. Dr Preston asks: What do my patients think about colds and fevers and how do different generations view their ailments?

Helman (1978) studied beliefs about illness in relation to changes in body temperature. He collected information by interviewing patients, district nurses, receptionists, and general practitioners in Stanmore, a suburb of London. He then generated a model which explained local beliefs about causes and remedies and studied their relationship to the beliefs and behaviour of the doctors.

Helman (1978) differentiated between the views of patients born before

World War II and those born during or after the War. Older patients categorized infectious disease according to their sensation of temperature. If they felt cold, they classified themselves as having 'chills' or 'colds'. If they felt hot they described 'fevers'. An extra dimension concerned the presence or absence of fluid. A temperature change could be accompanied by a dry condition. If an abnormal amount of fluid was felt to be within the body, for example, phlegm, or emerging from it, for example urine, the condition was described as wet. So four basic categories emerged: conditions that were cold and wet or cold and dry; and conditions that were hot and wet or hot and dry (see Table 8.1).

Table 8.1. *Categories of infection*

Wet or dry	Temperature	
	Hot	Cold
Wet	Hot, wet	Cold, wet
Dry	Hot, dry	Cold, dry

Chills occurred mainly below the waist and colds above it. The area was known to be damp and dangerous and changes in environmental temperature might bring on colds. People were responsible for protecting themselves by dressing up warmly and avoiding draughts and damp. Colds occurred when people exposed themselves to these hazards; for example, going out after a hot bath or with damp hair. Treatment was your own responsibility and remedies called for adding heat—hot drinks, hot water bottles, and a warm bed.

Fevers, on the other hand, were attributed to 'germs', 'bugs', or 'viruses'. They were transported by people and the victim was felt to be blameless. The majority of fevers were related to the presence of excess fluid and they were more severe, long lasting, and potentially dangerous. These beliefs related to expectations placed on the doctor. Patients sought fluid remedies to flush out a feverish infection. They wanted to know if an affected child should mix with other children. Since the advent of antimicrobial agents they expected specific drugs to kill the germ *in situ*.

Helman (1978) suggests that since World War II and the introduction of antibiotics the germ theory has come to account for several conditions on the 'cold' side of the classification. This has led to more frequent concern about the danger of mixing with others and increasing demand for 'anti-germ drugs'. The general practitioner, Helman points out, stands at the interface between medical models and lay beliefs about illness. The process of negotiation about therapy may result in the doctor becoming a source of folk remedies. For example, liquid is thought to wash out a feverish cough. Millions of gallons of cough mixture are prescribed annually. Folk models, he suggests, exert a powerful effect on the prescribing habits of many general practitioners.

Who are the lay experts and what do they think?

People in Wincampton do not move house frequently, so many extended families, which include three generations, are registered with Dr Preston. They sometimes express concern about a relative in the consultation. He realizes that families discuss their symptoms among themselves and consider causes and remedies for them. Because women tend to nurse the sick at home, their opinion and judgement is most often sought. Older women have more experience and are often regarded as community experts. He knows that the presence or absence of a grandmother and the advice she gives will often influence a young mother in her decision to consult him about her own health or that of her children. It would be interesting to know more about the views of these lay experts.

Blaxter (1983) interviewed 46 grandmothers in their homes. Her respondents lived in the city. They were in the semi-skilled or unskilled classes and they were not geographically or socially mobile. The interviews were relatively unstructured, taking the form of one- to two-hour conversations. Initial 'trigger' questions were used and a standard set of topics raised.

Blaxter (1983) found that certain diseases were seen as things, 'an arthritis', 'the whooping cough'. These types of diseases were seen as familiar, like old friends. Other diseases, like cancer or Parkinson's disease, were never preceded by a definite or indefinite article. They were alien and imposed on the body from outside. Diseases such as cancer and tuberculosis were generally named with no discussion of causation.

The women were able to discuss the cause of other diseases, particularly those which were regarded as old friends. By far the most common causal category was infection. The second most common cause was ascribed to heredity or familial tendencies. They described diseases running through families and favoured explanations which reinforced the picture of a long-term family identity.

The women recognized that disease was not mono-causal and connected together health events to create a logical sense of continuity in their lives. They felt that the diseases they experienced were not random. They believed that their childhood experiences, their pregnancies and deliveries, their work and environment, and the illnesses they suffered were all connected. The women drew on ideas derived from their family, neighbourhood, health professionals, and the media. By constructing chains of causality, they meaningfully linked together what they had experienced to create a continuous sense of individual and family identity.

Illness and responsibility

Dr Preston has noticed a wide variation in his patients' ideas about illness and their expectations of him. Despite severe symptoms, some patients do not want to bother him. Other patients bring minor complaints in the hope that he has a remedy. He is troubled by the morbidity statistics from general practice (RCGP, OPCS, and DHSS 1982) which show that working-class mothers bring their children to the general practitioner less frequently for immunization and preventive services, and wants to increase their involvement in preventive care. He asks: What do young mothers believe the causes of illness are? Can their beliefs be related to past experience or future behaviour? Are other factors like education and housing important in explaining patients ideas and behaviour?

Pill and Stott (1982) studied the concepts of illness causation and responsibility held by 41 young mothers in Wales. They identified the wives of skilled manual workers between 30–35 years of age who lived on an estate in Cardiff. The women were visited and semi-structured interviews undertaken.

The interviewer asked the women what they thought the main reasons for illness were and divided the responses into two broad categories. Some individuals tended to regard the causes of illness as internal; illness came, for example, as a result of being run down, neglecting oneself, or from a poor diet. Other women tended to regard the causes of illness as external to the individual. In this category they included environmental factors such as germs and family susceptibility. The former group were likely to stress individual hard work, good food, and positive mental attitudes when comparing their health with that of their grandparents' generation. The latter group saw improvements in health as being due to better medical services and better medicines.

The researchers related their findings to previous work by Rotter (1966) on locus of control. Rotter proposed that people develop generalized expectancies in learning situations as to whether success is dependent on their own behaviour or whether it is the result of luck, chance, or powerful others. He found that those who have a generalized expectancy or belief in internal control perceive events as contingent on their own behaviour. Those who have a generalized expectancy or belief in external control perceive actions which follow on their own as more likely to be due to chance, powerful others, or as unpredictable, owing to the complexity of the forces surrounding them.

Rotter (1966) proposed that a generalized expectancy or belief regarding the nature of the causal relationship between one's own behaviour and its consequences might affect a variety of behavioural choices in a broad band of life situations.

Pill and Stott (1982) divided their respondents into those who stress external factors and those who stress individual behaviour. They also grouped the women according to educational level and according to whether they were owner-occupiers or council tenants. Those who had more education and were home-owners were more likely to stress that individual behaviour caused illness. Those who had less education and who were council tenants were more likely to stress that only external factors were important.

Patients' beliefs and preventive action

These studies suggest that individuals combine lay and expert beliefs with their own idiosyncratic interpretations. Patients impose meaning on their experiences and connect them in an attempt to construct a coherent picture. Beliefs are different in different generations and between different social classes.

Lack of choice in many working-class lives may promote fatalistic views. In cross-sectional studies such as these it is difficult to test what comes first, beliefs or behaviour. Do beliefs cause behaviour or are they merely consequences of it? In the context of a particular life history, it seems likely that both situations occur in a continuous process:

Experience ⟶ beliefs ⟶ behaviour

In practice, Dr Preston is concerned about the possible relationship between fatalistic views among some working-class patients and their low uptake of preventive services. Can beliefs be related to preventive action? What instruments are available to measure this?

Pill and Stott (1987) subsequently developed a salience of life-style index which can predict a relationship between certain beliefs and uptake of preventive health procedures. The pilot phase of their study has already been described. It involved recording what range of life-style factors women mentioned spontaneously in the course of more general discussion about illness causation and responsibility.

They then administered a semi-structured schedule interview to 204 mothers, either classified in the Registrar General's social classes IV and V, or similar women who were not classified as they were single or unemployed. Procedures were established to achieve inter-rater reliability. The investigators asked open-ended questions about illness causation and prevention and awarded points for any mention of diet, exercise, smoking, drinking, etc. in the replies. They also recorded selected items of preventive behaviour like the timing of first antenatal visit during the last pregnancy.

They found that the group who showed a commitment to the importance (salience) of life-style choices in the prevention of disease were associated with those who in fact made use of preventive health checks. In other words there was a significant correlation between the measure of attitude towards prevention and the behaviour consistent with it.

Pill and Stott (1985) stressed that it would be misleading, however, to dichotomize people into two groups, life-stylists and fatalists. It is likely that nearly everyone accepts the view that illness is caused by factors outside individual control. Those who emphasized internal control did not reject causal theories like germs or heredity that would be classified as outside individual control. But these respondents stated that individual action can additionally contribute to the likelihood of falling ill. Using the salience of life-style index, they found that life-stylists hold more complex models of illness causation.

The investigators applied the methods of social science in the context of general practice. They have looked for associations between social characteristics, beliefs and attitudes, and health behaviours. A range of measures have been developed to identify clusters of beliefs and attitudes. But they stress it would be rash to overemphasize the predictive value of any of the measures so far developed—the relationship between attitude, beliefs, and behaviour is by no means straightforward. Collaborative research of this kind can contribute none the less to increased doctor–patient understanding and perhaps in the long run to increased uptake of preventive health care.

Screening and behaviour

In the previous study the researchers demonstrated a relationship between patients' beliefs about disease and their uptake of preventive services. Dr Preston is not only concerned with primary prevention, but also with screening to detect risk factors like high blood pressure. Before he embarks on a screening programme he asks: How will the detection and labelling of patients as hypertensive affect their behaviour?

A team at McMaster University (Taylor *et al.* 1981, Macdonald *et al.* 1984) prospectively investigated the effect of screening for hypertension on absenteeism at a steel mill in Hamilton, Ontario, Canada. A random two-thirds (5400) of male employees were screened. Two-hundred-and-forty-five men met the criteria for hypertension, 230 entered the trial, and 208 were followed-up over four years. Seventy men already knew they had hypertension when the trial began.

The researchers found that, in the year prior to screening, patients aware that they were hypertensive exhibited twice as much illness absenteeism as the unaware group. After screening, the men identified and labelled as hypertensive exhibited an 80 per cent rise in illness absenteeism in the follow-up year. The most startling rise in the year following screening was among men who did not comply with prescribed therapy. Their absenteeism actually increased fivefold. Although absenteeism did not rise significantly among compliant men in the first 12 months, it rose two to four years after the screening programme.

The researchers found that absenteeism was unrelated to the degree of hypertension, whether or not patients were placed on treatment or whether or not they achieved blood pressure control. In addition, the investigators related the effect which absenteeism had on income. Prior to screening, unaware hypertensives were earning slightly more than the normotensive control group. Five years following screening, those labelled hypertensive were earning significantly less than the same control group.

The investigators suggest that labelling a person hypertensive may lead to a change in his self-perception of health. The result is that at least some patients are more ready to adopt the sick role when minor illness occurs. Consistent with this labelling hypothesis are the findings that patients previously aware of their hypertension had significantly higher illness absenteeism to begin with and that previously unaware patients experienced a sharp increase in absenteeism when they were told that they had hypertension. In this study, screening was undertaken at the place of work. This facilitated the collection of data about absenteeism. Treatment was undertaken either at work or separately by the doctors in the community. There is some evidence from the UK Medical Research Council trial (Mann 1981) that the primary health-care team can co-ordinate screening and follow-up in such a way as to mitigate the adverse effect of labelling. This is a potentially promising area for action research.

Perceptions about chronic disease

In becoming aware of an asymptomatic condition, a patient's self-perception and behaviour may change. Patients react even more strongly when they develop recurring symptomatic conditions like seizures and are given the diagnosis of epilepsy.

Scambler and Hopkins (1980, 1986) identified a sample of 94 adults with epilepsy, who were registered with five London group practices. They visited the patients in their homes and undertook standardized interviews. Most respondents said they were extremely upset, even resentful, when they were informed they had epilepsy. Most felt that the doctor's diagnostic utterance had in a sense made them into epileptics. Uncertainty about the diagnosis and the patients' alarm often led them to try to negotiate for a less-threatening diagnosis.

Only one-third of the respondents could give details of one incident when they suspected another individual of stigmatizing them for having epilepsy. But 90 per cent of the patients made a general and unprovoked reference to epilepsy as a stigmatizing condition.

The patients' feeling of shame and fear of being stigmatized often led them to conceal their condition and, where possible, to pass as normal. Sixty-one per cent had never disclosed their condition to a boyfriend or girlfriend, and only 13 per cent always did so. Thirty-three per cent had made a full disclosure of their condition to their partner before marriage, while 31 per cent made no disclosure whatsoever before marrying.

The fear of being stigmatized also led individuals to conceal the diagnosis from their employers. Of 40 people who had had two or more jobs after the onset, 22 (55 per cent) had never disclosed their epilepsy. Eleven (28 per cent) had specifically informed their employers. Seven of these informed employers before starting work, two because of a form which enquired about epilepsy and five voluntarily. The people who volunteered the information tended to suffer from more frequent seizures.

The investigators suggest that those who are diagnosed as epileptic develop a special view of the world in which the fear of being stigmatized predominates.

This leads them to conceal their condition from others and to attempt to pass as normal. Whilst this approach reduces the chance of discrimination against them, it may also reduce their opportunities in the context of personal relationships and the employment market. The feeling of stigma precedes and may be more disruptive than any actual stigmatization they experience.

What are the implications of these studies?

Individuals combine lay and expert beliefs with their own idiosyncratic interpretations. Each patient imposes meaning on his experience and connects his experiences in an attempt to construct a coherent picture. Beliefs are different in different generations and between different social classes. The lack of choice in many working-class lives may promote fatalistic views, but these beliefs may become stable and significantly affect behaviour with regard to the preventive services which are available. Patients may respond to diagnostic labels in a way that has not been anticipated or intended. The fear of stigma which attaches to some diagnostic labels has social repercussions which profoundly affect some patients' lives. Not only do patients incorporate expert opinion, but general practitioners also incorporate lay views. Knowledge of this research increases the doctor's understanding of his role.

With this broader frame of reference, general practitioners may wish to learn more about patients' ideas in the process of the consultation. To what extent does this already occur? Tuckett *et al.* (1985) analysed 405 consultations recorded by 16 general practitioners. One-half of the doctors were selected because they had a reputation for being good communicators and had responsibility for teaching communication skills. The investigators found that in 8 per cent of consultations doctors made some active effort to invite patients to volunteer or to elaborate on their ideas. However, in 70 per cent of consultations no invitation was made or no interest expressed in listening to patients' ideas. When patients expressed ideas which appeared to disagree with doctors the investigators recorded that doctors often interrupted or changed the subject. In view of their role as experts in the community, it is surprising to find that women were twice as likely to have their ideas evaded by the doctor. The patients were subsequently interviewed in their own homes. Patients whose ideas had been inhibited or evaded could not recall or understand key points in the consultation as well as those who had been encouraged to express their ideas, and they were less committed to their doctor's advice.

Clearly patients' ideas, concerns, and expectations are crucial to their understanding of health and their use of health services. Pendleton and a group of general practitioners in Oxford (Pendleton *et al.* 1984) have developed exercises to help doctors discover and integrate patients' ideas with their own in the process of the consultation. They propose a reactive educational model in which doctors respond to patients' ideas, concerns, and expectations with individual tailored explanations and information (see Fig.

8.1). It would be interesting to measure the extent to which these educational techniques can be acquired by doctors. Pendleton *et al.* (1984) and Tuckett *et al.* (1985) suggest that more sharing of ideas increases patients' recall, satisfaction, and commitment to plans made in the consultation.

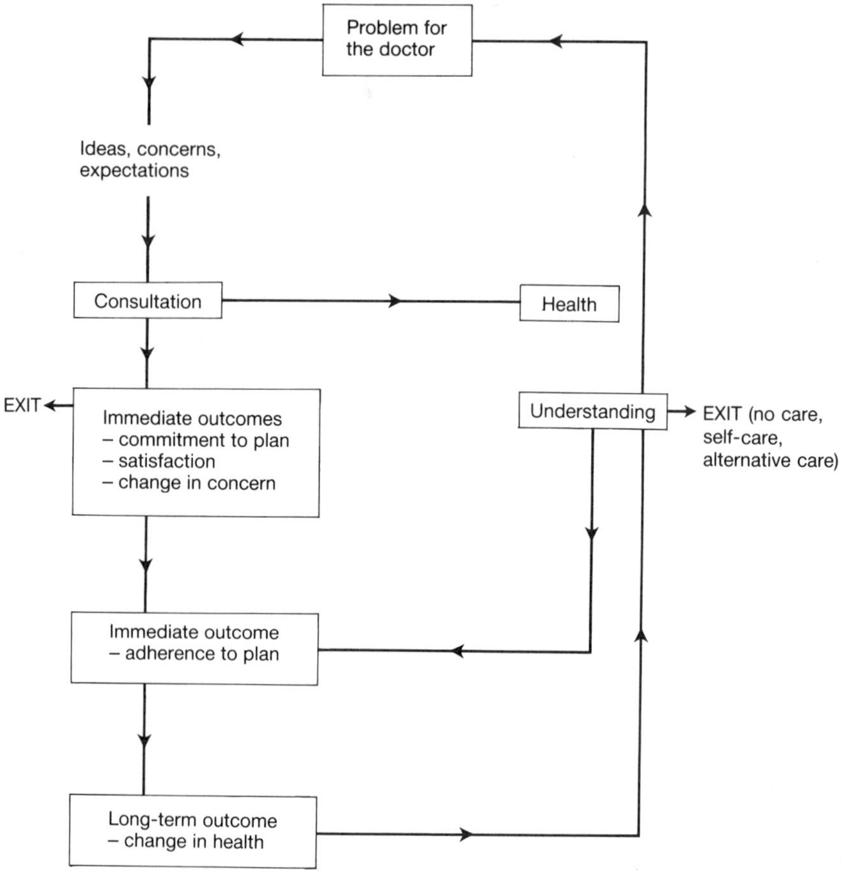

Fig. 8.1. The cycle of care (from Pendleton *et al.* 1984).

CONCLUSION

The studies described in this chapter indicate the complex nature of research which is concerned with exploring patients' beliefs about health and their use of health-care resources. It is important that Dr Preston should be aware of these complexities, and it is likely that he will feel able to investigate these aspects of his patients' behaviour only with help from behavioural scientists. As he becomes more involved in elucidating the behaviour of his patients, he may venture into this field and seek co-operation and funding for this type of research.

REFERENCES

Blaxter, M. (1983). The causes of disease—women talking. *Social Science and Medicine* **17**(2), 59–69.

Helman, C. G. (1978). 'Feed a cold, starve a fever'—folk models of infection in an English suburban community and their relation to medical treatment. *Culture, Medicine and Psychiatry* **2,** 107–37.

Macdonald, L. A., Sackett, D. L., Haynes, R. B., and Taylor, D. W. (1984). Labelling in hypertension: a review of the behavioural and psychological consequences. *Journal of Chronic Disease* **37**(12), 933–42.

Mann, A. H. (1981). Factors affecting psychological state during one year on a hypertensive trial. *Clinical and Investigative Medicine* **4**(3/4), 197–200.

Pendleton, D., Schofield, T., Tate, P., and Havelock, P. (1984). *The consultation—an approach to learning and teaching*. Oxford University Press.

Pill, R. and Stott, N. C. H. (1982). Concepts of illness, causation and responsibility: some preliminary data from a sample of working class mothers. *Social Science and Medicine* **16**(1), 43–52.

Pill, R. and Stott, N. C. H. (1985). Choice or chance: further evidence on ideas of illness and responsibility for health. *Social Science and Medicine* **20**(10), 981–91.

Pill, R. and Stott, N. C. H. (1987). Development of a measure of potential health behaviour: a salience of lifestyle index. *Social Science and Medicine* **24**(2), 125–34.

Royal College of General Practitioners, Office of Population Censuses and Surveys, and Department of Health and Social Security (1982). *Morbidity Statistics from General Practice*. Socio-economic Analyses. Studies on Medical and Population Subjects, No. 46. HMSO, London.

RCGP, OPCS, and DHSS (Royal College of General Practitioners, Office of Population Censuses and Surveys, and Department of Health and Social Security) (1986). *Morbidity statistics from general practice. Third National Study*, 1981–1982. HMSO, London.

Rotter, J. B. (1966). Generalised expectancies for internal versus external control of reinforcement. *Psychological Monographs* **8**(1), 1–28.

Scambler, G. and Hopkins, A. (1980). Social class, epileptic activity, and disadvantage at work. *Journal of Epidemiology and Community Health* **34,** 129–33.

Scambler, G. and Hopkins A. (1986). Being epileptic—coming to terms with stigma. *Sociology of Health and Illness* **8**(1), 26–43.

Taylor, D. W., Haynes, R. B., Sackett, D. L. and Gibson, E. S. (1981). Longterm follow-up of absenteeism among working men following the detection and treatment of their hypertension. *Clinical and Investigative Medicine* **4**(3/4), 173–7.

Tuckett, D., Boulton, M., Olson, C., and Williams, A. (1985). Meetings between experts—an approach to sharing ideas in medical consultations. Tavistock Publications, Andover, Hants.

9 How important is mental illness?

Deborah Sharp

Dr Preston is aware that many of the patients who consult him are sad or distressed by social and personal relationship problems. It is often difficult to know where to draw the line between a normal response to the 'ups and downs' in life and mental illness. He would like to be able to look more objectively at the amount of mental illness presenting in the practice and compare different methods of management. He recognizes the difficulty of defining such physical problems as hypertension or asthma. The definition of mental illness is clearly far more difficult and demands different epidemiological methods.

THE SIZE OF THE PROBLEM

Psychiatric disorders in the community, and in general practice in particular, have received a great deal of interest in recent years (Jenkins and Shepherd 1983), and they are best researched in an epidemiological context. This allows the assessment of the distribution and correlates of the particular disorders in a population and can also shed light on aetiology, course, and outcome. Information on health service organization and planning may also result. It is widely believed that one-third of general practice consultations are for purely physical conditions, one-third are for purely psychological conditions, and one-third are for a mixture of both. Thus in 66 per cent of all doctor–patient contacts there is a psychological component. When one considers that 98 per cent of the population are registered with a general practitioner and that 60–70 per cent consult at least once in any year and 90 per cent in any three-year period, with an average list size of 2000 and a consultation rate of between two and four, every general practitioner is going to see a great deal of psychological illness. In fact it has been well established (Shepherd *et al.* 1966) that general practitioners come into contact with, and are responsible for treating, most psychiatric disorders and that only a very small proportion of the mentally ill who consult their general practitioner are referred on to a psychiatrist and even fewer are admitted to a mental hospital.

Table 9.1 compares general practitioner consultation rates for diagnosed psychiatric disorders with those for out-patient clinics, day-patient attendances, and rates of admission. The general practitioner rates are taken from the Third General Practice Morbidity Survey (RCGP, OPCS, and DHSS 1986). General practice consultations for identified psychiatric disorder outnumber psychiatric out-patient attendance by roughly 7:1 and psychiatric admissions by 70:1. This demonstrates just one of the reasons why primary care is of such great importance in the care of the mentally ill. All epidemiology requires 'case definition' and most disorders behave as continuously distributed variables. Thus the question to be answered is not 'Has he got it?', but 'How much has he got?' In psychiatry there is an even more fundamental problem—deciding what 'it' is. Unlike most other branches of medicine 'there is no observable or measurable physical representation of mental illness so that its presence is largely a matter of opinion' (Birtchnell 1974, p. 335). This problem is magnified in general practice for three reasons.

Table 9.1. *Comparative rates of attendance for different levels of psychiatric care (ICD-9 290–315) (rates per 100 000 general population, all ages and sexes combined, in 1981)*

General practitioner consultations*	Out-patient attendances†	Day-patient attendances†	Psychiatric admissions†
22 980	3532	4943	397

*Obtained from RCGP, OPCS, and DHSS (1986).
†Obtained from *The Facilities and Services of Mental Illness and Mental Handicap Hospitals in England, 1980–81*. Department of Health and Social Services. HMSO, London.

First, many patients with a psychological disorder only present with a physical complaint and do not consider themselves to be psychologically unwell. Second, physical and mental disorders frequently coexist, and there is good evidence that general practitioners frequently miss psychological disorders (Goldberg and Blackwell 1970), just as psychiatrists may miss a physical disorder. Third, many psychological disorders are connected with family problems and social difficulties and can only be understood in the context of this information. It is worth mentioning at this point that the psychological problems seen in primary care are not easily classifiable as mental illnesses according to schemes such as the International Classification of Disease, 9th Version (ICD-9) or even the International Classification of Health Problems in Primary Care, 2nd Edition (ICHPPC-2). For example, in primary care many disorders are regarded as either depressive or anxiety neuroses. This distinction indicates the appropriate drug treatment, but does not take into account more precise phenomenological features, concurrent physical disorders, or the social and behavioural aspects. Thus there is an a priori need to develop a multiaxial system of classification (Mann *et al.* 1981).

Diagnosis

Individual general practitioner's estimates of the prevalence of psychological disorder, even in their own practices, vary enormously (Shepherd *et al.* 1966).

In a study in 46 general practices in and around London he found rates ranging from 6 to 65 per cent. It is hardly likely that such variation is due to differences in patient populations—the figures say much more about the doctors than the patients. Overall, of some 15 000 patients 'at risk' during a 12-month period, about 14 per cent consulted their doctor at least once for a condition diagnosed as entirely or largely psychiatric in origin.

Studies such as these and others allow the construction of models to describe the nature of psychiatric disorder in the community and how this is reflected in the organization of care. The most well known of these models is that of Goldberg and Huxley (1980), who use the concepts of levels and filters whereby one has to pass through a filter to get from one level to the next (see Fig. 9.1). Level 1 refers to all psychological disorders in the community, a large proportion of which pass through the 1st filter into level 2 when the patient decides to consult the general practitioner. However, a great deal of this psychological morbidity is not recognized by general practitioners and so these people do not pass through the 2nd filter. Level 3 is therefore the 'conspicuous psychological morbidity', most of which will be treated by the general practitioner. A proportion, however, will be referred onto the specialist mental health services, i.e. pass through the 3rd filter into level 4, and an even smaller proportion will be admitted to hospital, i.e. pass through the 4th filter into level 5.

Level 1	Psychiatric morbidity in the community
	1st filter: the decision to consult
Level 2	Total primary care morbidity
	2nd filter: general practitioner recognition
Level 3	Conspicuous primary care morbidity
	3rd filter: the decision to refer
Level 4	All psychiatric out-patients
	4th filter: the decision to admit
Level 5	Psychiatric in-patients

Fig. 9.1. Goldberg and Huxley's (1980) model.

The enormous variation between general practitioners in rates of conspicuous psychiatric morbidity was mentioned earlier. What causes this difference in diagnostic ability? Goldberg and Huxley (1980) suggest that 'bias' and 'accuracy' are important factors in determining this variation. Bias is largely determined by factors such as personality, attitudes, and experience of the general practitioner, whereas accuracy correlates with the general practitioner's behaviour during the consultation.

Bias refers to an individual general practitioner's tendency to make (or not make) a psychiatric diagnosis and is the ratio of conspicuous to true morbidity

$(a+c)/(a+b)$ (Table 9.2). Thus general practitioners who make more psychiatric diagnoses than are confirmed by psychiatric assessment have a high bias, and vice versa. But even if a general practitioner is 'unbiased' $(a+c)=(a+b)$, it may not be that the general practitioner and psychiatrist identify the same patients as being ill. Thus one can also measure 'accuracy'—the degree to which the general practitioner and psychiatrist agree:

$$\frac{(a+d)}{(a+b+c+d)}$$

Dr Preston finds the Goldberg model very helpful in conceptualizing the

Table 9.2. *Relationship between general practitioners' and psychiatrists' assessment of presence or absence of a psychiatric disorder for a series of general practitioner attenders*

Psychiatrists' assessment	General practitioners' assessment	
	Present	*Absent*
Present	*a*	*b*
Absent	*c*	*d*

usual course of a psychological disorder, but he is still somewhat perplexed by how he can improve his own identification rate. He has read all about this 'hidden' psychiatric morbidity and wonders if:

(1) there are certain characteristics of these patients which lead to their diagnoses being missed;
(2) there are certain characteristics of the doctors which result in their not making the diagnoses;
(3) it matters at all, because he is not sure whether identification improves outcome.

The majority of general practice psychiatry deals with psycho-neurotic disorder in contradistinction to the formal mental health services who spend much more of their time dealing with mental retardation, dementia, the psychoses, personality disorders, alcoholism, and drug addition. Two early studies showed that these psycho-neurotic disorders can be divided into two groups—half are of brief duration (less than a year) and are probably related to environmental stress, and the other half are relatively long-standing and are associated with some degree of personality disorder (Kedward and Cooper 1966; Cooper *et al.* 1969). Mann *et al.* (1981) produced the only good study on the outcome of minor psychiatric morbidity in general practice, and found that, over a one-year period, one-third improved within the first six months, one-third had a variable intermittent course, and one-third had chronic persistent symptoms. Outcome seems to be poorly predicted by the actual symptoms and diagnosis. Factors such as initial severity of symptoms and the presence of social stresses are more likely to predict duration of illness.

Goldberg and Blackwell (1970) found that patients whose psychological problems remained 'hidden' from the doctor often presented their problem in terms of physical symptoms. They can be divided into two groups. The smaller of these had a new and often serious physical symptom (e.g. rectal bleeding) which produced understandable anxiety and distress. Here the presentation of the physical symptom is appropriate, but the associated psychological distress is missed. In the second group, patients present a trivial physical complaint or re-present with a chronic problem (e.g. low back pain)—the symptom is again taken at face value and the psychological/emotional reasons for the consultation ignored.

On the other hand, patients with a psychiatric disorder not only consult their doctor more frequently, demanding a high level of care, but there is also a real association of physical and psychiatric morbidity. Eastwood and Trevelyan (1972) demonstrated this association from a health screening survey in a London general practice. In addition to a battery of physical tests, each patient completed a 20-item questionnaire (taken from the Cornell Medical Index), and those whose scores suggested a possible psychological disturbance were interviewed, resulting in 8.2 per cent confirmed cases. When this group of 'cases' was matched with a control group, the former appeared to have a significant excess of major physical disease.

The non-recording of a psychiatric diagnosis is not confined to general practice. Patients with major physical illnesses in medical and surgical hospital beds often will not have their psychological distress detected by the doctors looking after them. The reasons are similar to those in general practice. How can the non-specialist psychiatrist make a reasonably confident diagnosis of psychological disturbance?

What can we measure?

When measuring psychiatric morbidity in a population, a commonly employed research strategy is the two-stage screening survey (Goldberg 1972). In the first stage, a large number of individuals are screened with a case-finding instrument (usually a questionnaire) to identify 'probable cases'. The second stage comprises an interview (by a psychiatrist) with these probable cases to confirm or deny their 'case status'. Clinical psychiatry, however, is both an ill-defined and a non-standardized process, attributes which make it unsuitable as an epidemiological research tool. The need to operationalize definitions of diagnostic categories, as has been attempted by Feighner *et al.* (1972), and by Spitzer *et al.* (1978) by means of 'Research Diagnostic Criteria', is a step in the right direction—i.e. of measuring reliability in psychiatric diagnosis. Apart from the problem of reliability, other issues arise when measuring psychiatric symptoms:

(1) Which symptoms should be measured?
(2) How should they be measured?
(3) What do the measurements mean?

The symptoms included in a case-finding instrument need to be chosen with regard to their 'specificity' for the disorder and their ability to discriminate between 'cases' and 'normals'. The number and severity of symptoms should be taken into account, as well as the time period over which symptoms are to be measured. The design of the questionnaire with regard to 'acquiescence set'—the tendency to agree or disagree with items irrespective of their content—and to 'social desirability set'—the tendency to agree with items that are regarded by the respondent as socially acceptable or desirable, and vice versa—is also important. And, of course, the score on the questionnaire must have a meaning.

The validity of the instrument can be considered in two ways: criterion-oriented validity, which compares the instrument with a generally agreed upon external criterion, and content validity, which asks the question 'Is the content of the instrument appropriate to the variable being measured (psychiatric symptoms)'? Goldberg (1972) distinguished two models for the meaning of the actual scores obtained:

(1) the pathology or severity model, whereby a high score indicates greater severity;
(2) the probability model, in which a high score equates with a higher probability of being a case.

The final problem to be considered is what threshold is to be used to define cases and non-cases. Since all case-finding instruments determine probability, there will always be some degree of misclassification, i.e. false positives and false negatives will arise. If prescriptive screening is the aim of the enquiry, it is important for all individuals at risk to be identified, and thus the proportion of false negatives must be minimized by selecting a low cut-off point.

The efficiency of a case-finding instrument, or screening test, is evaluated from its sensitivity, i.e. its efficiency in detecting true positives (cases) and its specificity, i.e. its efficiency in detecting true negatives (normals) (see Table 9.3). The case-finding instruments are usually 'pencil and paper' tests that may be given to the patients themselves, in order to detect those who are most likely to have a psychiatric disorder. In a general practice population, most such illnesses are anxiety or depression states and the screening tests are mainly concerned with the symptoms of these. None of them make diagnoses, but several will provide a profile of scores as well as an overall score indicating the probability that a disorder is present.

Table 9.3. *Efficiency of a screening test*

Criterion classification	Screening test classification: Positive	Negative	Totals
Cases	a	b	$a+b$
Normals	c	d	$c+d$
Totals	$a+c$	$b+d$	$a+b+c+d$
	Sensitivity $=\dfrac{a}{a+b}$		Specificity $=\dfrac{d}{c+d}$

Questionnaires

The General Health Questionnaire (GHQ) is the most widely used of these screening tests. It is available in versions as short as 12 items and as long as 60 (Goldberg 1978). The GHQ was developed primarily for use in the community as a screening test for non-psychotic disorders. It is both valid and reliable, with over 50 well-conducted validity studies now reported. The scoring is somewhat unusual in that instead of measuring frequency or intensity to rate a symptom, it asks the respondent to compare his present state with his usual state. Symptoms are only counted if the patient is experiencing them 'more than usual' or 'much more than usual'.

The threshold score on any questionnaire will be affected by the degree of concomitant physical illness; for example, in general practice settings, the best threshold on the 30-item GHQ (GHQ30) is usually 4/5, but for an in-patient on a neurological ward it may be 11/12. If the GHQ is to be used in routine clinical work, then the best threshold is usually that point where the probability of 'caseness' is 50 per cent. However, the percentage of patients with high scores must not be supposed to be the same as the probable prevalence of the illness. The positive predictive value of a test is the probability that those with scores above the threshold will be thought to be cases. This will be around 50 per cent for those who score at the threshold, but it rises with increasing score.

The original studies of Goldberg and Blackwell (1970) describing the GHQ's validity and reliability were followed by studies that (1) compared general practice attenders with a community sample (Goldberg *et al.* 1976); (2) estimated the prevalence of psychiatric disorder in certain groups (Hobbs *et al.* 1985; Ballinger *et al.* 1985); and (3) endeavoured to measure the 'hidden' psychiatric morbidity of general practice (Goldberg and Bridges 1987). In this last study (3), the GHQ increased the detection of psychiatric morbidity compared with the general practitioner and in some cases the score was of prognostic value.

Similar to the GHQ is the Symptom Rating Questionnaire (SRQ), a 20-item inventory developed for use in the Third World by the World Health Organization. A recent comparison between the GHQ12 and the SRQ in Brazil showed them to be equally useful. Scaled screening tests to detect specific symptoms are also available and can be used as general case detectors by adding the scaled scores together. The GHQ28 consists of four subscales—somatic symptoms, anxiety and insomnia, social dysfunction, and depression—and was devised by a principal axes analysis of the GHQ60. It appears to be at least as good as the GHQ30 as a case detector (Goldberg and Hillier 1979). The Symptom Check List (SCL-90) has up to nine subscales. It is popular in the USA but has a rather low positive predictive value.

There are also specific screening tests. Particularly well known are the ones used to assess depressive symptoms. The Beck Depressive Inventory (Beck *et al.* 1961) is well validated against the Hamilton Rating Scale for depression and consists of 13 questions, each with a four-item response scale (Hamilton 1960). The Leeds Scales (for depression and anxiety) consist of six questions each, with similar four-item response scales (Snaith *et al.* 1976). There are many other rating scale questionnaires which have been devised for measuring particular symptoms in different settings. In each case, before an instrument is used, it should be validated in a sample of the population for which it is intended so that an appropriate threshold is determined.

Chronic social difficulties—measuring their presence and effect

Chronic social difficulties, such as financial hardship, social isolation, migration, and low social class, have been shown to be associated with in increased prevalence of mental illness. Such illness has itself important social consequences, not only for the individual, but for the families and for society in general.

The early classical studies on schizophrenia showed that first admissions were more prevalent in the poor, socially disorganized inner city areas. Debate has continued on whether this was due to schizophrenics drifting into these areas as a result of their illness or whether the illness was precipitated by the adverse conditions encountered in such areas. The former is thought to be more likely, but the relationship for minor psychiatric morbidity is less clear. In 1969, Dohrenwend and Dohrenwend reviewed 44 studies which had attempted to determine the true prevalence of psychiatric disorder in the community; their most consistent finding was of an inverse relationship between social class and rate of psychological disorder. They concluded that psychological symptoms in a community were of two main types; those generated by social situations and those generated mainly by personality defects. Social dysfunction can be measured, but with difficulty. An instrument is required that is sufficiently comprehensive to assess all the important areas of social functioning, yet can be used by workers from different professions in both general practice and in community settings. The Social Assessment Schedule (Clare and Cairns 1978) attempts to fulfil these criteria.

Three categories of social behaviour are covered. The first, material conditions, attempts to assess objective social circumstances—finance, occupation, and housing. The second, social management, looks at how the individual manages his affairs, activities, and relationships, covering areas such as financial management, leisure and social activities, family and domestic relationships, and marriage. The third category, satisfaction, enquires about the respondent's attitude towards various aspects of his life situation, housing, marital relationship, etc. In summary, the individual's life is examined from three standpoints—what he has, what he does with it, and how he feels about it. The three categories are intended to be operationally independent and the scale is scored in an essentially negative fashion, measuring degrees of dysfunction and maladjustment. Inter-rater reliability is high.

Acute social difficulties, or life events, as precipitants of psychiatric morbidity have received much attention recently. Marriage, bereavement, moving home, and childbirth are typical of life events which are stressful to some individuals but not to others. Whilst the research evidence for a causal relationship between life events and depression is still conflicting, much work has gone into developing instruments for their assessment.

The Schedule of Recent Experience (Holmes and Rahe 1967) was, until quite recently, the most commonly used instrument in this area. A self-report questionnaire, it covers 44 events and the patient is asked to allocate a score to each in terms of the amount of social readjustment required. It has been criticized on the grounds that it is too vague in specifying the situations or events. Paykel *et al.* (1969) produced a similar schedule of life events, but their technique requires an interview, at which the presence or absence of an event in the last six months is noted as well as its severity and its independence with respect to the presence of any current mental illness. This schedule was used to show that a higher frequency of life events was found in schizophrenics prior to their illness and in depressed out-patients. The signal work in this field was conducted by Brown and Harris (1978) on women in South London. They showed that working-class women were more likely to develop depression in the face of adverse life events if they were vulnerable by virtue of:

(1) lacking an intimate relationship with a partner;
(2) having a number of children under the age of 14 living at home;
(3) losing one's mother before the age of 11;
(4) being unemployed.

The Life Events and Difficulties Schedule is a rigorous interview, enquiring about all aspects of a person's life and the events that have occurred in the previous 12 months. The threat implied by the event is measured from the contextual threat perceived by the woman and as assessed by the interviewer.

Evidence that there is a connection between inadequate social supports and psychiatric illness has now been obtained from several studies. Henderson e *al.* (1978) in Australia found that psychiatric patients had smaller social networks and less-effective interaction with the primary attachment figure than matched controls. In another study, they found that the presence of a loving, intimate relationship was negatively correlated with the presence of neurosis. The effect of social support on illness is not wholly understood, but it may act by decreasing the number of stressful life events encountered or by decreasing their impact. The Interview Schedule for Social Interaction was developed specifically for use in these studies in an attempt to examine not the relationships themselves, but the availability and adequacy of those provisions which one believes people obtain from them (Henderson *et al.* 1980).

The Social Support and Stress Interview (Jenkins *et al.* 1981) was devised to assess stresses and supports in a variety of different life domains—occupation, finance, housing, social life, marriage, and the family. A semi-structured interview explores each area to establish the material position and the advantages and disadvantages of the patient's circumstances. The extent to which circumstances within a domain are stressful or supportive are rated by the subject rather than by the interviewer.

Interviews

The main diagnostic tool in psychiatry is the clinical interview. For research purposes the interview should be structured to some extent to ensure the same range of enquiry in each case and to improve reliability. A number of reliable standardized interviews for use in the second stage of a study, to confirm (or not) psychiatric case status, have been developed in recent years. It is essential that the interview chosen for a particular research study is appropriate. Some of the earlier interview schedules were developed only for administration to psychiatric patients and are not really suitable for community surveys.

The use of operational criteria to enhance diagnostic reliability was discussed earlier (p. 104). In the USA, Spitzer *et al.* (1978) elaborated the original Feighner criteria (Feighner *et al.* 1972)—Research Diagnostic Criteria (RDC)—to apply to symptom information obtained in any clinical interview. They then designed a structured interview, the Schedule for Affective Disorders and Schizophrenia (SADS) (Endicott and Spitzer 1978), which enables the interviewer to obtain and rate information about clinical features during the whole episode of illness as well as during the current month. Although the SADS and RDC have been used in community samples and are reliable when used by non-clinical interviewers, they were devised mainly for in-patients and the reliability studies were performed using psychiatric patients.

The Present State Examination (PSE) was devised by Wing *et al.* (1974) at the Institute of Psychiatry in London. This is a very comprehensive interview and uses a flexible clinical method whereby the interviewer can vary the procedure according to the patient's symptoms. It was originally developed as a diagnostic tool, but a modified, shorter version has been produced for general population studies. There is an associated computer program (CATEGO) which incorporates the diagnostic rules and gives a CATEGO class and an ICD-9 diagnosis where appropriate. An eight-point index of definition (ID) can also be devised which comprises levels of certainty that a disorder is present, ranging from no symptoms at all (ID1) through threshold disorders (ID5) to definite cases (ID8). An individual who is ID5 or above can be assigned a CATEGO class and an ICD-9 diagnosis. However, for a symptom to be rated at all on the PSE it must be 'clinically fairly severe' and so subjects with lesser degrees of symptomatology may fall through the net.

The attributes of an interview for use in the primary care setting are that:

(1) it should be acceptable to individuals who may not see themselves as psychiatrically disturbed;
(2) the content of the interview should be appropriate to the types of psychiatric disturbance seen in the community;
(3) it should discriminate clearly between cases and normals, and between patients with different degrees of psychiatric disturbance;
(4) it should be as concise as possible, so that large numbers of patients can be studied;
(5) it should be reliable in the hands of different interviewers.

Probably the most useful community interview is the Clinical Interview Schedule which was devised initially to act as the second stage for case-finding in the GHQ validity studies and later for research purposes in general practice and community surveys (Goldberg *et al.* 1970). The schedule is divided into four sections. The first is unstructured and records briefly the patient's present and past medical history. The second part consists of a detailed and systematic enquiry about any psychiatric symptoms which the patient may have experienced in the previous week. The ordering of the questions was designed to provide a progression from those symptoms commonly encountered in everyday life to those which are more obviously morbid mental phenomena. The aim for each question is to establish the frequency, duration, and intensity of each symptom, which is then rated on a five-point scale. The third section of the interview is unstructured and collects information on personal and family history. The final section requires the interviewer to rate any abnormalities observed during the interview on 12 five-point scales. Thus a total of 22 ratings is made and an allocation of case status can be decided on the basis of three different ratings:

1. Diagnosis—according to ICD-9.
2. A symptom score based on the total weighted score (TWS), where
   $TWS = \sum R + 2\sum M$, and
   R = score for each reported symptom, and
   M = score for each manifest abnormality.
3. An overall severity rating (OSR) ranging from 0–4, where 0 represents no

psychiatric abnormality and 4 is a psychiatric disorder requiring admission to hospital.

A case is most often defined as an OSR $\geqslant 2$. This interview is very reliable and has been used in many community studies in the second stage of the case-finding procedure.

CONCLUSION

This chapter has presented a bewildering array of methods of measuring psychiatric morbidity in the primary care setting. Dr Preston's original anxiety that he may be missing a good deal of his patients' psychological illness has been confirmed. He is now aware, however, of the fact that some patients are much more at risk of psychiatric illness than others—those with major physical morbidity, chronic social difficulties, and recent adverse life events. He also knows that women are at much greater risk than men, and that being separated or divorced also increases risk. Unemployment may also be a risk factor for psychiatric illness. But how many of these symptoms really constitute a definable psychiatric disorder and what are they a case of?

Is it a 'life problem' rather than a mental illness? This is an extremely important question to answer, especially in general practice, when a decision to treat or not to treat has to be made. This problem has been made more difficult in recent years by the fact that people are more likely to bring to the doctor matters which would not previously have been regarded as within the doctor's domain. By evaluating more rigorously, by whatever method, the presence or absence of key psychological symptoms, their intensity and duration, the general practitioner can investigate the incidence and prevalence of psychiatric morbidity in his practice. By the use of well-validated questionnaires he can identify groups of patients who can be followed up over a period of years to study the natural history of psychiatric illness or can be submitted to randomized controlled trials of alternative methods of treatment. Dr Preston may feel that it is easier to measure the outcome of the management of hypertension, diabetes, or asthma by the use of a sphygmomanometer, haemoglobin A estimates, or measurement of peak expiratory flow. He must accept, however, that psychiatric illness forms an important part of his workload and that it is helpful to be aware of methods which may be used to measure the prevalence of these disorders and the outcome of their management.

REFERENCES

Ballinger, C. B., Smith, A. H. W., and Hobbs, P. R. (1985). Factors associated with psychiatric morbidity in women—a general practice survey. *Acta Psychiatrica Scandinavia* **71**, 272–80.

Beck, D., Ward, G. H., Mendelson, M., Mock, J. and Erbaugh, J. (1961). An inventory for measuring depression. *Archives of General Psychiatry* **4,** 561–71.

Birtchnell, J. (1974). Is there a scientifically acceptable alternative to the epidemiological study of familial factors in mental illness? *Social Science and Medicine* **8,** 335–50.

Brown, G. W. and Harris, T. (1978). *Social origins of depression: a study of psychiatric disorder in women.* Tavistock Publications, Andover, Hants.

Clare, A. W. and Cairns, V. E. (1978). Design, development and use of a standardized interview to assess social maladjustment and dysfunction in community studies. *Psychological Medicine* **8,** 589–605.

Cooper, B., Fry, J., and Kalton, G. W. (1969). A longitudinal study of psychiatric morbidity. *British Journal of Preventive and Social Medicine* **23,** 210–17.

Dohrenwend, B. P. and Dohrenwend, B. S. (1969). *Social status and psychological disorder: a Causal Enquiry.* John Wiley, New York.

Eastwood, M. R. and Trevelyan, M. H. (1972). Relationships between physical and psychiatric disorder. *Psychological Medicine* **2,** 363–72.

Endicott, J. and Spitzer, R. L. (1978). A diagnostic interview: the Schedule for affective disorders and schizophrenia. *Archives of General Psychiatry* **35,** 837–44.

Feighner, J. P., Robins, E., and Guze, S. B. (1972). Diagnostic criteria for use in psychiatric research. *Archives of General Psychology* **26,** 57–63.

Goldberg, D. P. (1972). *Detecting psychiatric illness by questionnaire.* Maudsley Monograph 21, Oxford University Press.

Goldberg, D. P. (1978). *Manual of the General Health Questionnaire.* NFER, Windsor.

Goldberg, D. P. and Blackwell, B. (1970). Psychiatric illness in general practice: a detailed study using new methods of case identification. *British Medical Journal* **ii,** 439–43.

Goldberg, D. P. and Bridges, K. (1987). Screening for psychiatric illness in general practice: the general practitioner versus the screening questionnaire. *Journal of the Royal College of General Practitioners* **37,** 15–18.

Goldberg, D. P. and Hillier, V. F. (1979). A scaled version of the General Health Questionnaire. *Psychological Medicine* **9,** 139–45.

Goldberg, D. P. and Huxley, P. (1980). *Mental illness in the community: the pathway to psychiatric care.* Tavistock Publications, Andover, Hants.

Goldberg, D. P., Cooper, B., Eastwood, M. R., Kedward, H. B., and Shepherd, M. (1970). A standardized psychiatric interview for use in community surveys. *British Journal of Preventive and Social Medicine* **24,** 18–23.

Goldberg, D. P., Kay, C., and Thompson, L. (1976). Psychiatric morbidity in general practice and the community. *Psychological Medicine* **6,** 565–9.

Hamilton, M. (1960). A rating scale for depression. *Journal of Neurology, Neurosurgery and Psychiatry* **23,** 56–62.

Henderson, S., Duncan-Jones, P., McArley, H., and Ritchie, K. (1978). The patient's primary group. *British Journal of Psychiatry* **132,** 74–86.

Henderson, S., Duncan-Jones, P., Byrne, D. G., and Scott, R. (1980). Measuring social relationships—the Interview Schedule for Social Intervention. *Psychological Medicine* **10,** 723–34.

Hobbs, P. R., Ballinger, C. B., McClure, A., Martin, B., and Greenwood, C. (1985). Factors associated with psychiatric morbidity in men—a general practice survey. *Acta Psychiatrica Scandinavia* **71,** 281–6.

Holmes, T. H. and Rahe, R. H. (1967). The Social Readjustment Rating Scale. *Journal of Psychosomatic Research* **11,** 213–18.

Jenkins, R., Mann, A. H. and Belsey, M. (1981) Design and use of a short interview to assess social stress and support in research and clinical settings. *Social Science and Medicine* **3,** 195–203.

Jenkins, R. and Shepherd, M. (1983). Mental illness and general practice. In *Mental illness: changes and trends*, (ed. P. Bean), pp. 379–409. John Wiley, Chichester, Sussex.

Kedward, H. B. and Cooper, B. (1966). Neurotic disorders in urban practice: a three year follow-up. *Journal of the Royal College of General Practitioners* **12,** 148–62.

Mann, A. H., Jenkins, R., and Belsey, E. (1981). The twelve month outcome of patients with neurotic illness in general practice. *Psychological Medicine* **ii,** 535–50.

Paykel, E. S., Myers, J. K., Diendelt, M. N., Klerman, G. L., Lindethal, J. J., and Pepper, M. P. (1969). Life events and depression: a controlled study. *Archives of General Psychiatry* **25,** 340–7.

RCGP, OPCS, and DHSS (Royal College of General Practitioners, Office of Population Censuses and Surveys, and Department of Health and Social Security) (1986). *Morbidity statistics from general practice. Third national study, 1981–1982.* HMSO, London.

Shepherd, M., Cooper, B., Brown, A. C., and Kalton, G. (1966). *Psychiatric illness in general practice.* Oxford University Press.

Snaith, R. P., Bridge, G. W. K., and Hamilton, M. (1976). The Leeds Scale for the self-assessment of anxiety and depression. *British Journal of Psychiatry* **128,** 156–65.

Spitzer, R. L., Endicott, S., and Robins, E. (1978). Research diagnostic criteria. *Archives of General Psychiatry* **35,** 773–82.

Wing, J. K., Cooper, J. E., and Santonus, N. (1974). *Description and classification of psychiatric symptoms.* Cambridge University Press.

10 Can I prevent disease and disability?

Mike D'Souza

Having read in the preceding chapters the many different approaches to measuring the content and outcome of general practitioner care, Dr Preston decides that he might make a start by examining the preventive care carried out in his practice. This seems to him to be central to the epidemiological approach to primary care. If it is feasible he would like to institute changes in the organization of the practice so as to do more to prevent disease and disability. He decides, however, that this is something which must be thought through carefully in order to determine the pros and cons of any new initiative.

The present system of general practitioner care has evolved through responding to the demands of sick patients in a common-sense way, and by carrying out the routine preventive measures such as immunization and antenatal care that are widely accepted as useful. What is the evidence that doing more than this is worthwhile?

Furthermore, what are general practitioners' motives for doing more than just responding to their patients' requests for help. It has been suggested that many doctors unconsciously enjoy being 'rescuers' and therefore prefer their patients to be grateful 'victims'. This criterion might apply more forcefully if the general practitioner actively promulgates his medical usefulness without invitation. There might also be a danger that a too efficient health monitoring scheme might deter patients from retaining responsibility for their own health, and they might totally neglect making their own follow-up appointments if they are spoon-fed with computerized reminders for check-ups. Also, when it comes to some of the major health hazards such as cigarette smoking, surely the patients' motives are the key to the whole problem. So many people who have these dangerous habits do not seem to be ignorant, nor are they simply addicted. Rather, they seem to be deliberately taking risks in a semi-suicidal way. Is this urge to self-abuse sufficiently well understood to preach a simple good health message and expect it to be listened to?

Finally, it has been argued that a general practitioner could actually end up doing more harm than good. Patients might have to take time off work attending the surgery's health clinics; they might have their insurance policies loaded because of, for example, the creation of screening records of mildly raised blood pressures. Might not their surgical risks be multiplied by increased operations on benign tumours, etc. Also, there might be a loss of self-confidence and *joie de vivre* after unsuspecting patients are told they have early disease about which very little can be done. Indeed, some might feel persecution and guilt for not attending health programmes. Each of these bad outcomes might increase negative behaviour patterns and result in actual loss of health.

Against all these objections what can be said in favour of being comprehensive and positive about prevention? Perhaps the most important defence has to be that the general practitioner is continually being provided with opportunities to influence the natural history of disease. Simply viewing the business of general practice as responding to symptoms could result in most of the job being devoted to alleviating the aches and pains of self-limiting or chronic disorders, while symptomless life-threatening conditions were ignored. Even if there are uncertainties and dangers in preventive care, if general practitioners remain sensitive to these issues and concentrate on preventing death, disability, and discomfort it is possible to work out a rational plan that will encompass preventive care at many levels, which can be offered to those patients who wish to use it.

Epidemiologists have defined three levels of protection:

1. The first and most fundamental level of prevention is to prevent the actual inception of disease, so called *primary prevention*. The most important contribution to primary prevention in general practice is to ensure that all children in the practice are fully immunized by the age of 18 months. In addition, the general practitioner has an important role to play in health education in respect of diet, smoking, exercise, and dental caries.

2. The second level of prevention, *secondary prevention*, is concerned with the detection of pre-symptomatic disease by screening or case-finding in order to improve the chances of medical intervention being effective. This has been discussed in general terms in Chapter 3, but will be discussed in more detail in this chapter.

3. Finally, in *tertiary prevention*, there is the prevention of death and disability by the comprehensive and systematic care of established disease. Many would not consider this a proper level of preventive care, but merely normal good clinical practice or continuing care. However, setting up such special clinics to care for invited at-risk disease groups such as diabetics could be one of the activities considered by a practice as an extra contribution to preventive care.

Perhaps the most rational way of deciding upon what, if anything, can be done to improve the preventive activities of any primary care team is to review what can be done at each phase of a patient's life. However, it has to be recognized that the armamentarium for prevention in general practice is limited by the facilities available. These facilities are summarized below:

1. Patient contact (even without special invitation to screening it has been estimated that 70 per cent of a practice list will attend during one year, and more than 90 per cent in a quinquennium).
2. Immunization facilities.
3. Case-finding facilities (i.e. for doing extra tests on consulting patients).
4. Screening facilities (i.e. for inviting a target population to attend a special clinic for screening tests).
5. Preventive pharmacological intervention.
6. Preventive psychological intervention.
7. Health education materials.
8. Precept—the example of healthy living being set by the health-care team.

Dr Preston will need to consider how these facilities for preventive care could be expanded in his practice and how they might be applied to each phase in a patient's life to achieve adequate preventive care. The pros and cons for preventive care in each age group are described in detail in Appendix 10.1.

DR PRESTON'S PROBLEMS

In developing preventive care in his practice, Dr Preston needs to consider the current situation (e.g. What is the immunization status of the children in the practice?), how the current position can be improved (e.g. What are the barriers to complete immunization and what strategies will improve this situation?), and what changes are needed in the practice to provide a more prevention-orientated approach to medical care and what are the costs and benefits of such a programme. Some examples of the way in which various programmes may be developed are described.

Assessment of immunization status in a practice

The first requirement is to identify all children under the age of two years in the practice. This may be done with an age/sex register. If there is an attached health visitor in the practice, the names and addresses of children under two years may then be checked against the health visitor's records. There is normally a discrepancy between the names of the children on the practice register and those on the health visitor's register. This may be accounted for in two ways. The age/sex register depends for its accuracy on recording the new registrations in the practice and the notification of removals from the practice by the Family Practitioner Committee (FPC). The latter are usually several months out-of-date. The health visitor's records are updated through a network of communication between health visitors, which is much more accurate. In some areas, practices span different health districts. In this case the attached health visitor may only have accurate information for children in her own health district and will depend on notifications from adjoining health districts about immunizations carried out. Health visitors usually have detailed records of the immunization status of the children under their care. The checking of the immunization status of children registered with the practice but not supervised by the attached health visitor can be very time-consuming unless the health district maintain good records centrally.

When a practice does not have an attached health visitor, it may be more difficult to establish base-line data concerning the immunization status of children in the practice. If centralized records are held by the health authority then lists of children registered with the practice may be checked against these records. If these data are not held centrally, it may be necessary to check the records with all the health authority clinics in the practice catchment area.

If a practice holds its age/sex register on computer, it is usually possible to add to the computer register immunizations which are carried out at the practice and to print out the results. When a practice newly acquires a computer the provision of this resource may be undertaken as follows:

1. Develop an age/sex register.
2. Search the health visitor's records and programme the current immunization status of all children covered by these records into the computer.
3. Develop a routine for typing into the computer all immunizations carried out in the practice.
4. Obtain a print-out from the computer of the immunization status of all children under two years of age, registered with the practice, and identify those whose immunization appears to be incomplete.
5. Determine by letter, telephone, or home visit the immunization status of those who appear to be incompletely immunized. Some of these will have left the district; others will have been immunized at health clinics outside the district and this information will not have been provided for the practice. A variable number will not have availed themselves of the services provided and may be encouraged to complete their immunization programmes.

Parents' attitudes to immunization

In any study of this type a number of unimmunized children will be identified and the doctor may be interested to find out why this has occurred. A study by Morgan *et al.* (1987) was developed to answer this question on a district-wide basis in terms of measles immunization. They interviewed mothers at 13 and 20 months after the birth of their children. At 20 months they found that the most common reasons why the child had not received measles immunization was that the child had already suffered an attack of measles, that there was concern about the contra-indications to the use of vaccine, or that there was delay due to intercurrent illness. For doctors wishing to investigate the reasons for the lack of uptake of immunization in their practices this study provides a useful model of epidemiological investigation.

The development of a programme for cervical screening

A method of developing a cervical screening programme in general practice has been described (Ridsdale 1987) and this could be carried out in any general practice with minimal costs.

A two-partner practice serving a population of nearly 5000 people recruited a nurse/midwife and sponsored her training for the Certificate in Family Planning. A well woman clinic was started in which family planning, cervical screening, and antenatal services were provided by a doctor and the nurse working together. A poster was placed in the waiting-room to inform patients of this service.

A state-enrolled nurse was recruited for three months by the practice on a half-time basis. Using the age/sex register, the nurse identified women aged 36–60 years. Those who had undergone a hysterectomy were identified from the patient records and excluded from the population at risk. The records of the remaining eligible population were used to audit the number of women who had been screened for cervical cancer in the past five years. Two women were found to have had mild abnormalities with no follow-up. These women and the women who had not been screened in the past five years were sent a letter offering an appointment for screening with the practice nurse. Letters were sent out, starting with the oldest women and progressing downwards through the age groups. The number of women responding to the letter and the number attending for screening were noted. Abnormalities among the smears taken were recorded using a protocol to ensure adequate follow-up. The cost to the practice of the smear-taking and administration was estimated.

The audit showed that 70 per cent of the eligible population of women had been screened for cervical cancer in the previous five years. The percentage of women who had been screened was inversely related to age.

Of the women sent a letter offering an appointment for cervical screening, 63 per cent responded. On receiving the letter some women responded with the information that they had not had sexual intercourse and were not at risk from cervical cancer. These women are included among the refusals. Fifty-seven per cent of the women attended for a smear test. Of the 37 per cent of patients who did not respond to the letter some were subsequently found to have moved away. The proportion of patients who failed to respond varied between age groups and was highest in the group aged 41–45 years.

After the study, 87 per cent of eligible women aged 36–60 years in the practice population had received cervical screening in the previous five years.

Of the 110 smears taken from women attending after receipt of the first letter, 84 were normal, nine showed inflammation, ten showed mild dyskaryosis, and three showed moderate dyskaryosis. Smears from three patients showed marked dyskaryosis or cervical intra-epithelial neoplasia, grade III.

The cost of smear-taking and administration for the practice was approximately £600. The FPC reimbursed the practice through item-for-service payments and 70 per cent reimbursement of salaries for practice staff. Those costs to the National Health Service (NHS) included smear-taking, administration, and laboratory processing, and the Department of Health and Social Security estimates the cost of this to be £4–£15.40 per smear taken, with a mean of £10. The total cost of the call programme to the NHS is therefore likely to be approximately £1100.

The three patients with marked dyskaryosis were treated by laser therapy and cone biopsy; the cost of this is difficult to estimate. However, if they are prevented from developing cervical carcinoma they will have cost approximately £366 per case identified. Had their disease progressed to clinical carcinoma, treatment would certainly have cost more. The benefits in terms of human suffering, although difficult to measure, must also be taken into account.

Assessment and intervention in the elderly

A detailed description of a method of developing a screening service for visual problems in the elderly has been described in Chapter 3. Similar protocols have been developed for carrying out regular assessments of disability and need in the elderly. Hendrikson *et al.* (1984) described in detail a system of assessment and intervention in a randomly selected group of patients aged 75 years or over. As compared with a control group, they were able to demonstrate a reduction in the number of admissions to hospitals and nursing homes and a reduction in the number of deaths. Significantly fewer emergency calls were received from the intervention group compared with the controls.

Multiphasic screening in general practice

Private medical services have strongly recommended multiphasic screening as a cost-effective method of prevention. The average general practitioner may be concerned about the possible benefits of introducing such a scheme. As compared with studies of immunization, cervical cytology, and assessments in the elderly, the costs and benefits of multiphasic screening in apparently healthy populations are difficult to measure in a single practice. An example of a study in which two large group practices co-operated with the Department of Epidemiology at St. Thomas's Hospital Medical School is described to illustrate the methods employed and the results obtained.

This survey was the South East London Screening Study carried out by Holland *et al.* (1977). The design of this study illustrates some of the problems likely to be encountered in this type of work; it is perhaps worth examining in detail as its methods, as well as its conclusions, have a direct bearing on judging the work of screening in general practice.

Two large suburban London group practices participated, with a combined total list size of 20 000. The two practices were not neighbouring because there was considerable difficulty in recruiting practitioners with sufficient motivation and organization to collaborate with a proper controlled study. Age/sex registers in these study practices were used to identify a population of men and women aged 40–65 years in 1966. This population was 7229 and it was randomly split into two groups; an intervention screening group and a control group. The medical records of both groups were studied for the year prior to entering the study to establish initial similarity; thereafter, consultation rates by cause, sickness certification, hospitalizations, and deaths were continuously collected for the purpose of comparison. The intervention screening group was invited to two successive 'multiphasic' screenings at two-year intervals. This screening comprised a detailed health questionnaire, blood tests, and physical tests such as blood pressure, PEFR (Peak Expiratory Flow Rate) audiometry, and electrocardiographs. There was also a physical examination by their own general practitioner extended to cover in more detail any abnormalities discovered by the screening.

After five years, nearly 25 per cent of the study population had been lost due to death or migration from the area, so it was decided to bring the study to a close by organizing a terminal survey screening of both the screening group and the control group so that direct morbidity comparisons could be made.

The results of this study were uniformly negative and, despite a great deal of effort, no measurable differences in mortality or morbidity were found. However, despite its scale, the study population was nearly five-times too small to be expected to show differences in death rates. Also, although many things were screened for and many abnormalities were found, very little medical intervention occurred as a result of the screening, chiefly because the doctors felt that there was little they could do about many of the abnormalities found at screening.

The general conclusions drawn from this study were that such comprehensive screening is at present unlikely to produce significant improvements in health. Screening was, however, popular with patients, and some 70 per cent of those invited did attend. In general, however, less-ambitious, limited target screening have produced more promising results (e.g. see Lannerstad *et al.* 1977). It is clear that intervention should be aimed at much younger age groups for such risks as smoking and hypertension. A full review of the literature on the value of the periodic health examination has been reported by the Canadian Medical Association (1979).

INTRODUCING SCREENING AND CASE-FINDING IN GENERAL PRACTICE

This is concerned essentially with identifying vulnerable groups in the general practitioner's community and ensuring that certain observations and tests are carried out on these individuals. The vulnerable groups may include the entire population in certain age groups, such as pre-school children, or selected groups such as sexually active women in predetermined age groups. In general practice, the problem is concerned with developing methods of identifying these populations, developing records which ensure that the observations are made and recorded on these populations, and developing methods of ensuring that, when abnormalities are detected, appropriate action is taken.

The introduction of computers to general practice has greatly facilitated this activity. They can be used to maintain age/sex/morbidity registers as described in Chapter 2. They can also be used to collect and organize information and to produce output which summarizes the findings. They can be programmed to alert the doctor to the need for repeat examinations or for management according to a predetermined protocol. Two examples are presented of ways in which the computer can be used, first to collect the information from patients newly registering with the practice, and second to develop a call and recall system for a vulnerable group of patients.

Some of the major problems of constructing a computerized age/sex register have already been solved in certain areas of the UK where it is possible to copy the computerized data held by the FPC with a suitable practice computer. Many commercial programs are now available to keep this practice listing up to date and to add variable amounts of information to the basic register of names. Such age/sex registers are, of course, essential office information that can form the basis of screening and recall systems on all patients or on selected subpopulations. However, it is essential to take independent advice before purchasing software or hardware in such a rapidly changing field as computing. Some practices will still prefer to construct their own age/sex register from the notes they hold. It is usually important to have both a double entry system to stop inaccuracies and a system capable of continuous updating. However, because changes are occurring in the list population every day, some of which are not notified to anyone, it is quite impossible to be 100 per cent accurate. In a practice of 8200 in Kingston, Surrey, for example, the age/sex data accurately obtained by double entry from the notes were compared with a computer print-out of the local FPC list and there were 240 minor inaccuracies in the FPC data, such as addresses, etc., but only 57 missing registrations were discovered (M. Tooley, private communication). So many doctors may consider it worthwhile to accept the FPC's lists.

In this same Kingston practice, a computerizable system for case-finding (ALIS; Appointment List Information System) has been used for over 10 years. This enables the consulting doctors to record, on a specially constructed encounter form, case-finding for smoking and hypertension, with additional space for immunizations and diseases of research interest (in this practice's case they take a special interest in auditing their asthma patients) (see Appendix 10.2). The system operates by the doctors asking each consulting patient at the start of each calendar year whether they have the conditions selected for case-finding. In the case of hypertension, blood pressure is measured and, if raised, the reading, together with a recall time, is written down on the form. With smokers, a record is also made of current cigarette smokers together with whether health education has been given. Should the surgery be very busy, or the case-finding be missed because it is emotionally inappropriate, etc., it can easily be deferred for a subsequent visit and the fact that case-finding has been done or not recorded in the notes. The information is transferred from the ALIS form onto the computer, which can be programmed to print out appropriate recall letters. The system can also be operated manually by a clerical worker with responsibility for organizing the recall system.

In developing the preventive role of his practice, Dr Preston is going to have to face up to the question of whether or not to try to persuade his partners to buy a computer. In doing this he will have to use arguments which prove that computers can not only improve the care of the patients, but improve the income of the practice. The following facts may help him to develop these arguments:

1. Most practices fail to provide systematic care for all patients who are registered with them. With a computerized age/sex register, an increased income can be obtained from undertaking all those services that attract a fee, such as cervical screening and immunization. Thus more efficient care can generate financial benefits for doctors and health benefits for patients.
2. Tedious jobs, such as writing repeat prescriptions and reminder letters, are done much better by machines. In the case of the former activity, automatic checks on abuse of the system can be incorporated into the programs as well as warnings on drug interactions and advice on how to use the medication.
3. The costs of the computer, including the essential insurance of hardware and software support and staff training, can be offset against tax as a part of practice business expenses.
4. The price of powerful machines is now quite acceptable to medium-sized practices.
5. There is good advice on choice of systems available from a number of independent sources, such as the Royal College of General Practitioners.
6. There are subsidiary uses for a computer, such as:
   (a) assistance in book-keeping and preparing letters;
   (b) word-processing for the practice that produces articles, etc;
   (c) statistics packages for the practice that conducts research;
   (d) interactive diagnostic and treatment programmes for practices that are interested in advancing the use of computers in clinical medicine, e.g. expert systems.

Dr Preston could argue that the quality of his practice in general could be greatly improved by the sensitive introduction of more efficient and comprehensive prevention. A computer could, if carefully chosen, considerably help this aim.

REFERENCES

Brown, G. W. and Harris, T. (1978). *Social origins of depression: a study of psychiatric disorders in women*. Tavistock Publications, Andover, Hants.

Curtis-Jenkins, G. H., Collins, C., and Andrew, S. (1978). Development surveillance in general practice. *British Medical Journal* **1,** 1537–40.

Canadian Medical Association Task Force (1979). The periodic health examination. *Journal of the Canadian Medical Association* **121,** 1193–1254.

Dales, L. G. *et al.* (1973). Multiphasic check-up evaluation study 3,—outpatient clinical utilisation, hospitalisation and mortality experience after seven years. *Preventive Medicine* **2,** 221–35.

Hakama, M. (1982). Trends in the incidence of cervical cancer in the Nordic countries. In *Trends in cancer incidence causes and practical implications*, (ed. K. Magnus), pp. 279–93. Hemisphere Publishing Corporation, Washingon DC.

Hendriksen, C., Lund, E., and Stromgard, E. (1984). Consequences of assessment and intervention among elderly people: a three year randomised controlled trial. *British Medical Journal* **289,** 1522–4.

Holland, W. W. *et al.* (1977). The South East London Screening Study Group. A controlled trial of multiphasic screening in middle age: results of the South East London Screening Study. *International Journal of Epidemiology* **6**(4), 357–63.

Lannerstad, O., Sternby, N. H., Isacsson, S. O., Lindgren, G., and Indell, S. E. (1977). Effects of a health screening on mortality and causes of death in middle aged men. *Scandinavian Journal of Social Medicine* **5,** 137–40.

Morgan, M., Lakhani, A. D., Morris, R. W., Dale, C., and Vaile, M. S. B. (1987). Parents' attitudes to measles immunisation. *Journal of the Royal College of General Practitioners* **37,** 25–7.

Patrick, D. L., Peach, H., and Gregg, I. (1982). Disablement and care: a comparison of patient views and general practitioner knowledge. *Journal of the Royal College of General Practitioners* **32,** 429–34.

Ridsdale, L. L. (1987). Cervical screening in general practice: call and recall. *Journal of the Royal College of General Practitioners* **37,** 257–9.

Russell, M. A. H., Taylor, C., and Baker, C. D. (1979). Effects of general practitioners' advice against smoking. *British Medical Journal* **2,** 231–5.

Smithells, R. W. *et al.* (1981). Vitamin supplements and neural tube defects. *Lancet* **2,** 1425.

Wilcox, R. G., Mitchell, J. R. A., and Hampton, J. R. (1986). Treatment of high blood pressure—should clinical practice be based on results of clinical trials? *British Medical Journal* **293,** 433–7.

APPENDIX 10.1: OPPORTUNITIES FOR PREVENTIVE CARE IN EACH AGE GROUP

Pre-conception

The most obvious opportunity for taking effective preventive measures before conception is presented when couples come asking for genetic advice. Here, appropriate referral for specialist genetic counselling and/or conducting simple tests for genetic markers are the obvious courses of action. However, in recent years there is a growing body of opinion that routine advice should be given to all couples who are intending to have families. Based on available evidence, there would seem to be at least three useful messages. The first is the common-sense advice that there are great advantages in planning babies, such that they are spaced and conceived at a time when the family is ready to cope with them. Second, there should be clear warning of the hazards to the early embryo of drinking an excess of alcohol, smoking cigarettes, and consuming drugs, or, indeed, of being on extreme slimming diets, and ensuring that all women are immune to rubella before conception. Third, there is advice on the value of adequate nutrition during early pregnancy, particularly the value of vitamin B supplements in those at risk for neural tube defects (Smithells *et al.* 1981). In certain cultures, such as the Greek Cypriots, where there are arranged marriages there is a known high risk of conditions such as thalassaemia. It is possible to get screening performed on both parties prior to any arrangements of marriage being agreed. Occasionally there will be a known risk of hereditary disorders among some patients and it will be important for doctors to inform them of this and to arrange for them to be appropriately screened by a clinical geneticist, particularly now that gene probes are becoming available for couples at risk for cystic fibrosis and Huntington's chorea.

If the general practitioner is to make any systematic contribution to prevention in pre-conception counselling, it is necessary to develop a routine which acts as an *aide-mémoire* for this activity. The majority of prospective mothers use a variety of methods of family planning before undertaking a pregnancy, and this presents an opportunity to apply preventive counselling. Many doctors have developed flow charts for family planning. Spaces can be included in these to remind the doctor to check on such things as smoking habits, alcohol ingestion, history of hereditary disorders, and rubella immunization status. Such reminders help to develop a positive approach to pre-conception counselling.

The foetus

The principle activity of general practice in caring for the foetus is in routine antenatal care. It is important that antenatal clinics should be organized to provide adequate time for high-risk parents. At a physical level this is concerned with identifying anaemia, urinary tract infection, and pre-diabetes in early pregnancy, and later the early identification of pre-eclamptic toxaemia, retarded foetal growth, and potential abnormalities. There is a very important part to be played in emotionally supporting the family during the time of pregnancy, and the continuity of care provided by the general practitioner is of great value in this. Recent work has also shown that psycho-social support can prevent disease in the mother and during the time of giving birth. No new screening seems necessary here as antenatal care is well established.

Neonates

The screening of neonates is generally a hospital activity, but sometimes the diagnosis of phenylketonuria, hypothyroidism, or hypoglycaemia and other biochemical disorders are made in general practice. Certainly the issue of whether developmental clinics should become a routine part of all general practices is worthy of debate. The evidence that it is a way of preventing a great deal of disease has not been satisfactorily provided, but those practices in which such developmental clinics are run do have an excellent start in forming good relationships with their patients (Curtis-Jenkins 1978). This is not least because patients are seen at times when there is no overt disease. A routine examination at six weeks of age is carried out by many general practitioners. On this occasion, the doctor is concerned with identifying any special problems the mother may be experiencing, detecting any gross abnormalities of motor function, including congenital dislocation of the hips and cardiac murmurs, ensuring the testes are in the scrotum, and monitoring weight gain and head circumference.

Toddlers and infant schoolchildren

Simply because very young children present with such a large number of viral infections during this time, many general practitioners will have the opportunity of seeing most of those in their practices. There is no evidence that adding systematic screening or any other intervention can prevent long-term problems. The development of a series of routine visits at seven months, two years, and three-and-a-half years, however, does ensure that certain parameters are checked at certain intervals, the most important being weight, vision (including the presence of squint), hearing, speech development, musculo–skeletal abnormalities, and the child's behaviour in the context of the family. Confirmation that all immunizations are properly completed can be integrated into this system and should ideally be a joint activity with the health visitors. Practices with age/sex registers and computers can develop programs to monitor immunization status. Many health authorities are now in the process, however, of instituting both data bases and follow-up systems. This could improve immunization uptake without general practitioners needing to set up their own schemes.

The extension of baby clinics to cover toddlers is widely practised, but some would argue that the yield of unsuspected disease from these clinics over and above that detected by normal practice is insufficient to justify them. More importantly, those patients who do *not* attend such clinics are often those most at risk of both physical and emotional problems. The running of clinics to identify non-attenders may in itself be worthwhile, provided that resources are available to chase up these non-attenders. Serious social hazards such as child abuse and neglect are best sought out during the normal clinical process.

Junior schoolchildren

There is in the United Kingdom an established school medical service and most general practitioners are reluctant to duplicate this. A wide range of problems such as disorders of special senses, undescended testes, cardiopulmonary diseases, and skeletal abnormalities may be diagnosed early in this group, but there is little evidence that special efforts to screen in general practice at this age are justified.

Secondary schoolchildren and teenagers

One of the important characteristics of this age group, in common with young adults, is that they are relatively infrequent attenders at the surgery, so screening might be more productive than case-finding. However, relatively few preventable problems go unnoticed by active youngsters. More important in this age group is to deter teenagers from starting unhealthy habits such as smoking, heavy drinking, and drug-taking, but the role of the family doctor in this important area has not been fully developed. Although a good deal of research into the factors associated with smoking in children has been carried out, few successful programmes of intervention have been reported. It seems likely that action in schools and changes in government policy, such as banning cigarette advertising, is more likely to be effective than action through the primary care team. The research of Brown and Harris (1978) relating depression in women in later life to traumatic events during puberty, such as bereavement and parental divorce, indicates that there may be a particularly vulnerable group of teenagers in every general practice. The development of ways of identifying these individuals in primary care and of providing counselling opportunities for them with members of the primary care team may be a useful prevention of subsequent emotional damage. Perhaps the most important proven preventive health measures that the general practitioner can undertake in this age group is to ensure that all teenage girls are immunized against rubella.

Young adults

This age group is generally the most healthy but is starting out on life-time habits that can be seriously damaging to health. The most important of such habits is smoking, and systematic anti-smoking health education has been shown to produce modest benefits (Russell *et al.* 1979). Other health risks which may develop insidiously in young adult life include obesity, problem drinking, promiscuity, genital infection and pre-malignant cervical changes, and a variety of cardiovascular risk factors including raised serum cholesterol and hypertension. A major decision which has still not been settled despite extensive research is at what age to start case-finding for hypertension and at what levels to institute treatment. Summarizing the findings of a variety of studies, Wilcox *et al.* (1986), after reviewing the trial literature, conclude that there is no appreciable benefit to an individual patient from treating a diastolic pressure of less than 100 mmHg, phase V.

Increasing evidence is accumulating for the value of screening for pre-malignant changes in the uterine cervix (Hakama 1982). A consensus is forming that the screening should be undertaken from the age of about 20 years in sexually active women and repeated at three-year intervals.

One activity which many general practitioners are concerned with is family planning, and this may usefully be linked with instruction on breast self-examination, advice on obesity, the identification of sexual and marital problems, and the dangers of promiscuity.

An important cause of death and disability in this age group is accidents on the road or during sporting and recreational activities. There is no evidence that the primary care team can make any useful contribution to reducing these hazards by health education, but the general practitioner should always bear these in mind in consulting with his patients.

Middle age

About 70 per cent of patients in this age group attend at the surgery each year and the potential for case-finding for hypertension, smoking and early cancer is correspondingly increased. In the USA, physicians advise a routine sigmoidoscopy to detect bowel cancer (Dales *et al.* 1973). The evidence supporting this screening procedure is not strong and few general practitioners in the UK would ever consider this.

General advice to encourage positive health and well-being, such as developing habits of regular exercise and a sensible diet, could be provided in a more systematic way, but epidemiological knowledge of the value of this is incomplete and over-dogmatic statements as to the advantages or hazards of many life habits are open to debate. For example, it has only recently been recognized that vigorous squash-playing in the over-40s is more dangerous than beneficial. Similarly, cycling in busy city centres may be beneficial as an exercise but dangerous because of the risk of road traffic accidents. Advice about the importance of developing at least two activities or interests that will extend beyond retirement may protect against emotional morbidity in old age and could be routinely given, but there seems little extra to be done at this time that should not have commenced earlier.

Retirement and old age

The principal issue to be considered in this age group is screening for those disabilities that prevent the enjoyment of retirement. There is evidence that general practitioners know too little about the problems of everyday living of their disabled patients (Patrick *et al.* 1982). This is particularly unfortunate where this prevents adjustments and modifications to the home being provided that can improve the quality of life. However, one of the commonest disabilities is deafness and a surprising number of people with this do not wear their hearing aids when issued with them. In fact, it seems that most aids, including even walking-sticks, are seen as stigmata of old age that can as readily remove social dignity as they support physical function. However, the idea of routinely asking those patients who have obvious disability such as strokes or osteoarthritis about their problems with daily living should form part of routine clinical care and may be carried out by health visitors and community nurses as well as by general practitioners.

Since the aim of medical intervention in old age is focused on the quality of life, the issue of being able to discuss the prospect of death in order to prevent anxieties of pain and isolation during the process of dying may also be a significant part of preventive care of some patients. It is much more likely that patients will be able to tolerate discomfort, disability, and even death if they have a composed philosophical outlook. However, judging from the psychiatric morbidity among doctors themselves, many feel that finding such an outlook is no easier for them than for their patients. Nevertheless, a caring management of death with clinically effective pain-relief can always be promised and this in its own right will be of considerable benefit.

APPOINTMENTS LIST INFORMATION SYSTEM (A.L.I.S.) "CASEFINDER"

DATE day / month / year

CLINIC 1 Morning 2 Baby 3 Antenatal 4 Evening 5 Research

DOCTOR 1 JB 2 JK 3 MD 4 SH 5 Other 6 Trnee 1 7 Trnee 2

INSTRUCTIONS:– TICK / IF YES, LEAVE BLANK IF NO BUT *ALWAYS* TICK LAST COLUMN. RECORD EACH CASE-FINDING IN MEDICAL NOTES WITH FULL DATE. E.G. SCREENED 01/04/87.							**ASTHMA?** Recurrent Wheezy Bronch.		**HYPER-TENSION?** Use Diastolic BP PhV "Disappearance" BP today		**SMOKING?**				**TICK** here means all blank cols are NO
TIME	SURNAME	FORENAME	SEX M = 1 F = 2	YEAR OF BIRTH	SERIAL NO. Not Reg'd. = 00000	ALREADY ASKED ONCE THIS YEAR (see notes)	NOW? i.e. <1 yr. having Symps.	on Drugs	NOW? i.e. <1 year B.P. ABOVE 99mm	on Drugs	Cigarette Smoker in past Year	Health Education given today	RESEARCH	IMMUNISATIONS If Needed R for Rubella F for 'Flu jab	↓

11 Would it be better if I moved?

Brian Jarman

Towards the end of his day, feeling himself rather overworked and disillusioned with his partners, Dr Preston may be wondering whether he would be better off moving to a practice in another area. This may lead him to consider the complex relationships between levels of morbidity and mortality, social factors, and service provision (in terms of primary and secondary health care) and also to consider the relationship between 'need' (however that is defined) and demand for health services. Although Dr Preston may not be thinking of these things in such precise terms, considerations of this type should influence his thinking.

HEALTH STATUS AND SOCIAL FACTORS

Rates of illness and death—morbidity and mortality rates—are commonly used as indicators of ill health. The concept of good health as a sense of physical, psychological, and social well-being is not one which is easily amenable to quantification, and it has been necessary to make do with these cruder measures of morbidity. Doctors are usually far from the idea of thinking about psychological and social well-being, let along measuring them, when they talk of health and ill health in its narrow sense.

Mortality rates are relatively easy to record and are very complete because death registration is compulsory. Death is an event that is easy to define even if the diagnosis recorded on the death certificate may be uncertain. There is the additional advantage with death certification that occupation is recorded when deaths are registered and hence death rates may be related to occupationally defined social classes. However, a general practitioner will have, on average, only about 25 deaths of patients on his list every year, whereas he will have around 7000 consultations with his patients. Therefore, death rates are very crude measures of his workload.

General practice morbidity surveys

Workload for general practitioners in a community will be indicated to a certain extent through records of the diagnoses made at consultations. National general practitioner morbidity surveys give an idea of recorded morbidity and, as practices are increasingly making use of computer systems, some of which can be used to record diagnosis, it can be expected that this type of morbidity information will become more routinely available. Because practices in the UK have registered lists of patients, consultations rates, the natural history of diseases, and workload can be calculated in relation to a defined practice population—a great advantage of the general practice system in operation in this country. If patients' addresses are postcoded, then recordings by a number of practices can be merged together on a geographical basis and the general practitioner recorded morbidity data for a particular area, such as an electoral ward (around 5000 people), can be estimated. Some of the weaknesses of general practitioner recorded morbidity were described in Chapter 2, but they are considered in more detail here and some possible solutions suggested:

1. The sheer volume of information to be analysed, and the virtual impossibility that an averagely busy general practitioner would be able to tackle this task himself, is a major problem. Nationally adopted computer programs are needed to perform these analyses and to produce results in a uniform manner so that they can be merged together and hence be of general as well as local use. The Joint Computer Group formed by the General Medical Services Committee of the British Medical Association and the Royal College of General Practitioners (RCGP) is studying this as well as the requirements of a morbidity recording code suitable for use in general practice.
2. It is difficult to define or code the content of a general practitioner consultation for computer analysis. Physical illnesses are easier to code than psychological or social problems and this is one of the issues that the Joint Computer Group is considering.
3. General practitioners see only a proportion of the illness in a community. Most people do not consult a doctor when they feel ill and may go first to a chemist rather than to a general practitioner.
4. Morbidity surveys are not necessarily representative of general practitioners as a whole. Attempts are made to take the practices which volunteer to do the recording from as wide a geographical distribution as possible, but some areas, such as London, tend to be under represented and there is still the problem that the practices are volunteers rather than randomly selected.
5. Conventionally recorded illness levels are not necessarily a good measure of workload or ill health in its wider sense. Psychological and social problems may cause much greater stress for a general practitioner than the physical illnesses that he has been taught how to deal with. Whether or not he is prepared by his training to deal with these problems, a general practitioner is probably the most accessible professional for patients to consult, and many problems having a psychological or social basis may be presented to him as physical symptoms which he cannot deal with adequately without attempting to unravel the underlying psychological or social causes. He may be relatively powerless to change these in comparison to his ability to take action for physical illnesses. For physical illnesses, even those for which there is no cure, he can often feel that he is doing something if palliative treatment or

investigations are needed, or he can provide comfort in his role as a doctor. How is it possible to measure the morbidity, taken in its widest sense, that social conditions and the consultations that they lead to, cause for the patient and the doctor?

6. Most general practitioner morbidity recording studies have not routinely recorded details of the social conditions of patients—such as household and family conditions like overcrowding, elderly living alone, single parent family, and so on. Health status and use of health services have been shown in population surveys to be related to these factors and it is therefore relevant to record them for individuals.

7. General practice morbidity data are based on a registered practice population rather than on a defined geographical area and it is difficult to relate these data to census data which are reported for groups of people in geographical areas. This difficulty could be overcome if the census data for patients registered with a practice were available to link with the morbidity data, but this is not possible for reasons of confidentiality. The general practitioner could record the data himself, but so far this has not been done. Alternatively, the data from different practices could be merged if the patients' addresses are postcoded, but the problem here is that complete coverage of the areas would be needed by all of the general practitioners involved and this is difficult to achieve.

The first two of these weaknesses can be overcome to a certain extent as computers become more sophisticated, the successive decennial editions of the International Classification of Diseases become more appropriate for primary care, and the RCGP's code is extended. In addition, the James Read code, which is adapted for computerization, allows actions taken, results of tests, and so on to be coded in addition to diagnoses. The last four weaknesses, however, will continue to pose problems. The extent of any error introduced by the third can be determined, to a certain extent, by comparison with the results from the General Household Survey, during which, for the last 15 years, a randomly selected sample of private households (reduced to about 12 000 in 1982) has been asked, among other things, about acute and chronic health problems in the two weeks preceding the survey. This is however only a small sample and it depends on self-reported illness and on the memory of the person being questioned. The great problem of the relationship between measures of morbidity and the actual workload or pressure on the services of general practitioners has only recently been tackled; this subject is dealt with later in this chapter.

Other morbidity measures

There are other measures of morbidity, all of which have a number of drawbacks. Illness certification records for payment of sickness and invalidity benefit because of sickness absence from work (forms Med 3 and Med 5) do not cover the whole population and are inaccurate, being used purely for the purposes of benefit payment. The Hospital In-Patient Enquiry is an approximately 10 per cent sample of non-psychiatric hospital deaths and discharges taken from hospital activity analysis data. These are not recorded with uniform accuracy by all district health authorities, apply to deaths and discharges and not to individual patients, and are obviously only applicable to hospital morbidity. Cancer registers only cover serious illness. Notifications of infectious diseases are notoriously incomplete.

Generally speaking, therefore, very reliable, objective, ongoing measures of the morbidity of the population are not available. Some routinely collected objective data, such as the proportion of low-birthweight babies and the proportion of those over 16 years of age who are temporarily sick or permanently sick or disabled, are available, however, but they give a very imprecise estimate of workload in general practice on the basis of which health care resources may be distributed. It is possible that a chronic illness question will be included in the 1991 census and thus give a more detailed measure of the geographical variations in morbidity.

Townsend (Townsend *et al.* 1986) suggested that the following measures might be used to estimate needs for care in populations:

(1) permanent sickness or disability data derived from the census;
(2) low-birthweight babies analysed by 'postcodes';
(3) still births and infant mortality as a combined rate;
(4) standardized mortality ratios (SMRs).

It has been shown that two social variables, unemployment and proportions of unskilled workers, explain nearly 80 per cent of the variation in SMRs up to the age of 65 in the district health authorities in England.

General practitioner workload or pressure on general practitioner services

With all this in mind and in order to have an idea about how social and other conditions affect general practice workload, questionnaires were sent to a randomly selected one-in-ten sample of general practitioners in the UK asking them to weight a number of factors according to the degree to which they considered that the factors increased their workload or pressure on their services when present in their area (Jarman 1983, 1984). The factors recorded were a series of thirteen social and eight service factors which an earlier survey had indicated were likely to be important. The general practitioners surveyed were asked to weight each factor on a scale of 0–9 in relation to the perceived importance of the factors in contributing to their workload.

The survey produced a 77 per cent response from the general practitioners to whom it was sent. In general, they gave much greater weighting to social rather than to conventional medical factors (except the level of psychiatric illness). The average weightings for each factor were very similar for general practitioners from all the 115 Family Practitioner Committees in the UK. The 'proportion of elderly people living alone' in each area was given the greatest importance of weighting (its average weighting was 6.62 ± 0.60 on the scale from 0–9). With this information, it was possible to construct a score based on the level of each of the social variables, taken from the 1981 National Census, in any area, each of these variables being weighted in accordance with the national general practitioner survey. Some of the variables and weightings derived from the general practitioner survey on a 0–9 scale are illustrated in Table 11.1.

Table 11.1. *Average weightings from survey of UK GPs of factors increasing their workload or pressure on their services.*

Variables	Weighting
Elderly living alone	6.62
Under 5s	4.62
Unskilled	3.74
Unemployed (% of economically active)	3.34
Single parent families	3.01
Overcrowded	2.88
Mobility—changing house within a year	2.68
Ethnic—New Commonwealth and Pakistan	2.50

These scores could then be summated to give a total score which may be claimed to reflect potential workload in general practice. The score was called the underprivileged area score or UPA score. It is a measure of the opinions of a national random sample of general practitioners of the degree to which the populations of various areas of the country are likely to increase their workload or pressure on their services. As such it is a census-based measure of general practitioners' opinions of potential workload related to their assessment of the morbidity, in the widest sense, which they see in the patients who consult them. It has the advantage over other measures of morbidity in that it is not related purely to physical illnesses. It is nationally applicable, based on uniformly collected information at the time of the national census, and can be applied to areas of various geographical sizes, each of which is built up of enumeration districts (which are the small areas covered by an enumerator who collects information for the census and covers about 150 families). It has the potential weakness that it is based on subjective estimates by general practitioners of the effects of the variables selected on their workload. The areas for which UPA scores have been calculated so far are illustrated in Table 11.2; these are shown tabulated by FPC in Appendix 11.1.

UPA scores and the related social data (as percentages of the resident population—except for unemployment, which is a percentage of the economically active) have been sent to a wide variety of organizations and individuals concerned with health and social services, including many general practitioners. The information can be used in the planning of services, as it gives an indication of the social conditions and potential workload in various

Table 11.2.

Area*	Approximate number in 1981	Approximate average population
Enumeration district (E & W)	112 000	430
Electoral Ward (E & W)	9300	5200
Local authority district† (E & W)	400	120 000
District health authority (E)	200	200 000
Family Practitioner Committees (E & W)	98	500 000
Regional health authority (E)	14	3 300 000

*E = England; W = Wales.
†Local authority districts may be grouped into 109 boroughs, etc.

areas. General practitioners have found that data based on the electoral ward are the most useful as their practice areas usually cover a few electoral wards and the boundaries of electoral wards are fairly well known. Computer programs are now available which can draw maps of various areas and shade them according to the levels of social conditions or UPA scores.

To test the validity of this method, blank ward maps were sent to local medical committees of five FPC areas and the general practitioners were asked to shade the wards black, grey, or unshaded according to the degree to which, in their opinions, the populations in their areas were likely to increase their workload or pressure on their services. The shading was based on the general practitioners' local knowledge and experience of the populations in their area and they were not given any census or other information other than the boundaries of the electorial wards.

Figure 11.1 illustrates the comparison between the maps shaded by the general practitioners and those constructed from the UPA scores. In the five FPC areas there was a good correspondence between maps shaded by the general practitioners and those constructed from UPA scores, with only 1.4 per cent of pairs of wards differing between the two sets of maps in areas where the general practitioners shaded complete wards.

A survey similar to that carried out with the national sample of general practitioners was done for a national sample of health visitors and for all community nurses in one district health authority. It was found, in general, that general practitioners and community nurses gave very similar weightings to each of the variables; that general practitioners and district nurses gave slightly higher weightings to the elderly; and that health visitors gave slightly higher weightings to the young and single parent families. Scores developed using community nurses' weightings of the census variables are very similar to those developed from general practitioners' weightings, and both groups give similar pictures of the geographical variations in scores.

Bradford UPA scores map

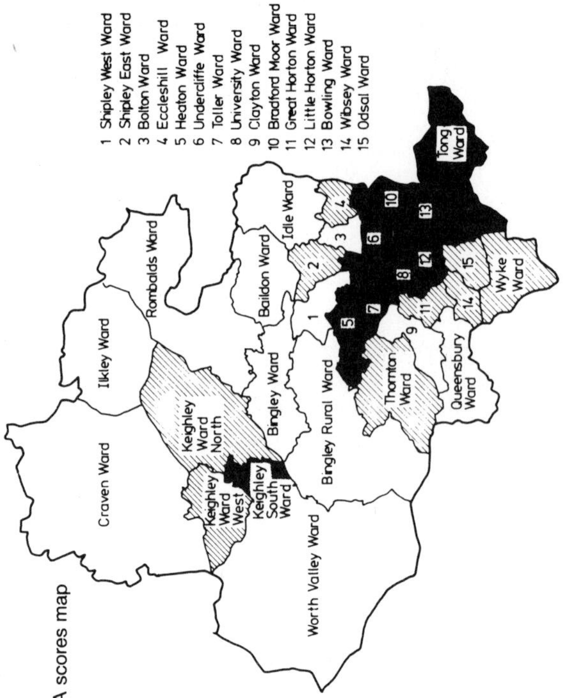

Bradford LMC map.

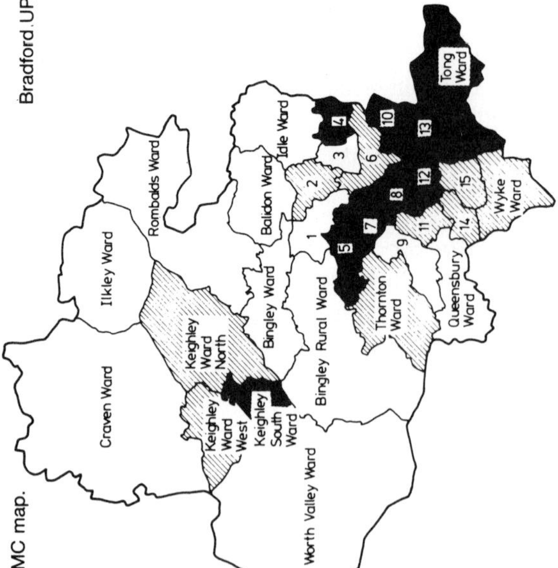

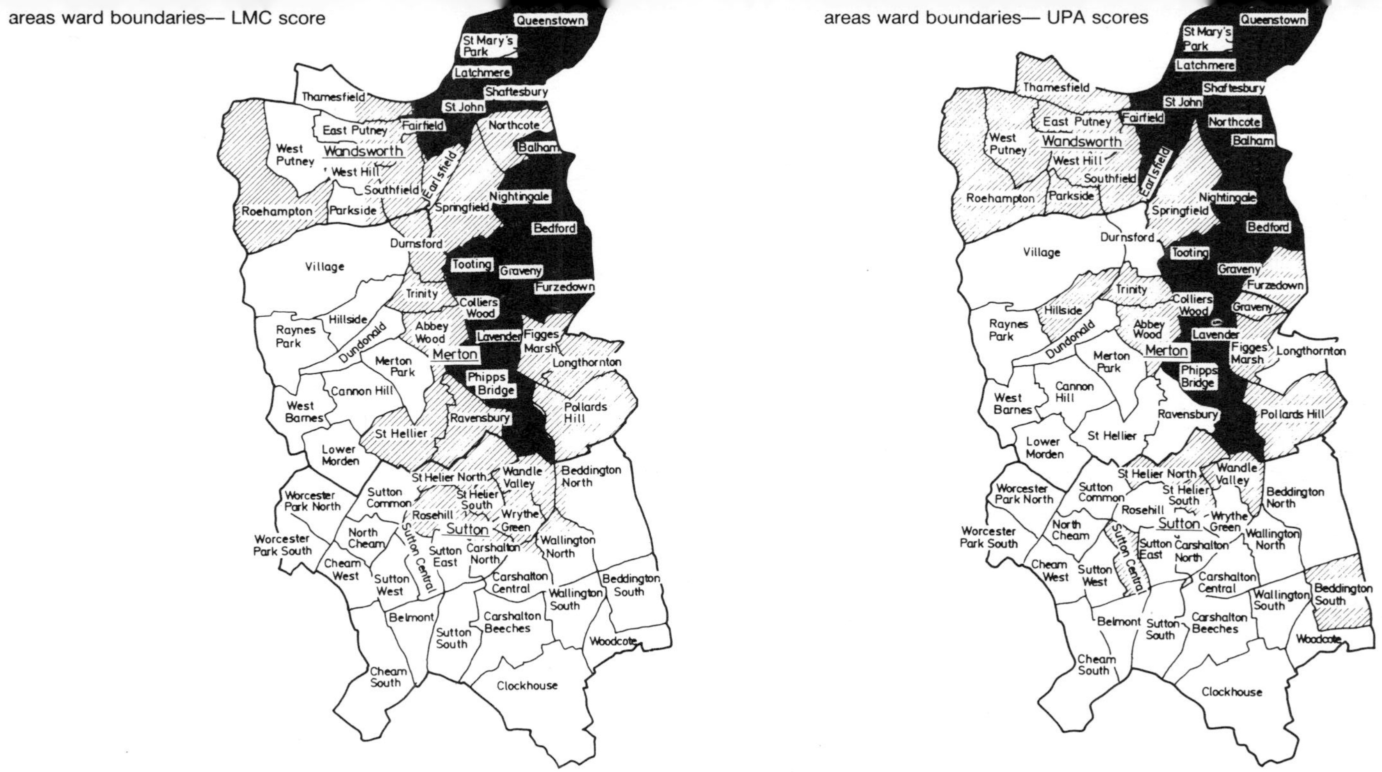

Fig. 11.1. Shading of wards according to increased workload or pressure on general practitioner services in four of the five (Northamptonshire too detailed to show) FPC areas by local medical committees (LMCs) and by UPA scores. Cut-off levels between the black (worst), cross-shaded (intermediate), and white (best) areas differ among FPC areas. (From Jarman 1984.)

UPA scores have been found to correlate strongly with other measures of morbidity, such as the proportion of low-birthweight babies in different areas and also with some service factors such as admission rates to hospital (after these have been standardized to allow for effects of age and sex). Individual social components of the score—unemployment, socio-economic grouping, overcrowding in households—are more strongly associated with standardized mortality ratios. The factors which are associated with higher usage of hospital services are those related to housing conditions and the care available to look after people at home, e.g. high proportions of elderly living alone, single parent families, and overcrowding of households.

Although based on subjective estimates of workload produced by a variety of demographic and social factors, derived from a postal questionnaire completed by a sample of general practitioners, UPA scores appear to be fairly robust (Charlton and Lakhani 1985) and to correlate with a number of other measures of workload. It is important to bear in mind that they may not necessarily correlate closely with workload as measured by consultation rates in general practice because they reflect not just the contact rate between doctors and patients but also the content and complexity of consultations.

Need and demand for health services

'Need' for health service may vary according to who is defining the need. Professionals—doctors, nurses, and so on—may consider that the need to reduce levels of morbidity and mortality is of paramount importance. Many developing nations have achieved remarkable improvements in conventional measures of health, e.g. reducing infant mortality rates and increasing life expectancy, often to levels approaching and sometimes better than those of developed countries. These improvements in health status have come largely as a result of public health measures, such as better sanitation, providing purer water supplies, and by a general improvement in nutrition and social conditions. Better education for women (who have most to do with the upbringing of children) seems to be of particular importance, as are campaigns to increase immunization levels and advice about treatment of diarrhoea and other medical conditions. Because the health element of these campaigns has been in the primary care and public health sectors, rather than in the relatively more expensive secondary health-care sector, the improvements have often been achieved at a remarkably low cost.

Planning primary health care

Health-care and social policy planners can be justifiably proud of reductions in morbidity and mortality, but patients themselves may have other concerns. They may find that they are treated in an impersonal way, with long waits to see their doctors and little or no continuity in the doctor–patient relationship. In developed countries, people may not appreciate the screening campaigns to detect hypertension or cervical cancer which their conscientious doctors may be carrying out if they are unable to see a doctor quickly when they feel they are ill—although they will justifiably be unhappy and angry if they develop an illness which their doctor could have prevented by screening. It is important that the patient's viewpoint is given the attention it deserves when planning services and assessing needs.

Administrators may be less worried about improvements in health status or providing a service responsive to patients' perceptions of their needs if the people who appoint and control them put the cost of the health service above other considerations. This may be a matter of national policy or the prevailing ethos of a health authority. In a system dominated by costly secondary care, these may be people of importance in providing that type of care. Although in these circumstances there will be attempts to achieve cost-effective secondary care by better management, it is difficult to cross the boundary between secondary and primary care (which is often less expensive). This conflict can cause low morale in both the secondary and primary care sectors. This stress is greatest in areas with higher UPA scores because they tend to be under financial pressures as a result of resource reallocation.

Other perspectives in evaluating general practice

Consultation rates and UPA scores are just two ways of looking critically at the content of general practice. Jarman (1981), in a study of Inner London general practices, described a variety of other measures of general practice, many of which may be derived from data currently available from FPCs. Some, which may be helpful in evaluating a prospective practice, are:

1. The cost of land and premises which may be used for the delivery of primary care and ways in which the cost/rent scheme may succeed or fail to compensate general practitioners' work in, for instance, urban centres.
2. The cost and availability of ancillary staff and the provision of premises to accommodate a primary care team.
3. The contribution which mileage allowances and dispensing fees may make to the practice income.
4. The difficulties and dangers in inner cities in providing out-of-hours care.
5. The mobility of the population which influences both the consultation rate and the content of the consultations.
6. The ease of access to hospital facilities, both for patients and for the educational needs of the general practitioner.
7. The relative attractions of a major city with its cultural facilities, as compared with a provincial town or rural area free from traffic congestion, parking problems, and violence, but perhaps providing relative isolation from colleagues, continuing education, and secondary medical care.
8. Opportunities for contributing to undergraduate teaching and vocational training.
9. Employment opportunities for a spouse and schooling opportunities for children.

It would appear that Dr Preston is somewhat unhappy in his present practice and suspects that the grass will be greener on the other side of the fence. Many of his problems may arise from his relationship with his partners or his expectations of general practice. In this chapter a number of ways of looking at the workload and content of general practice have been described and some of the other factors which may be considered in selecting a practice.

REFERENCES

Charlton, J. and Lakhani, A. (1985). Is the Jarman Underprivileged Area Score valid? *British Medical Journal* **209,** 1715–16.

Jarman, B. (1981). A survey of primary care in London. *Journal of the Royal College of General Practitioners*, Occasional Paper 16.

Jarman, B. (1983). Identification of underprivileged areas. *British Medical Journal* **286,** 2505–8.

Jarman, B. (1984). Underprivileged areas: validation and distribution of scores. *British Medical Journal* **289,** 1587–92.

Townsend, P., Phillimore, P., and Beatie, A. (1986). *Inequalities in health in the Northern Region.* Northern Regional Health Authority and University of Bristol.

APPENDIX 11.1 FPCS WITH HIGHEST AND LOWEST UPA SCORES

FPC	UPA Score
Highest	
1. City and East London	53.05
2. Camden and Islington	41.31
3. Lambeth, Southwark, and Lewisham	39.76
4. Manchester	37.73
5. Bradford	36.60
6. Kensington & Chelsea, and Westminster	33.95
7. Rochdale	26.45
8. Birmingham	25.65
9. Liverpool	25.61
10. Oldham	22.05
11. Newcastle Upon Tyne	20.85
12. Ealing, Hammersmith, and Hounslow	18.88
13. Kirklees	17.08
14. Calderside	16.14
15. Bolton	15.86
16. Salford	15.85
17. Wolverhampton	14.93

18. Sunderland	14.56
19. Coventry	13.96
20. Cleveland	12.80
Lowest	
79. Hillingdon	−11.98
80. Barking and Havering	−12.05
81. Oxfordshire	−13.01
82. North Yorkshire	−13.46
83. Stockport	−13.58
84. Hereford and Worcestershire	−13.86
85. Staffordshire	−14.00
86. Berkshire	−14.37
87. Kingston and Richmond	−14.42
88. Staffordshire	−14.50
89. Essex	−14.91
90. Gloucestershire	−15.61
91. Somerset	−15.87
92. Powys	−15.89
93. Buckinghamshire	−18.94
94. Dudley	−19.94
95. Warwickshire	−25.11
96. Bromley	−25.92
97. Solihull	−26.17
98. Surrey	−30.91

12 Common pits and how to avoid falling into them

David Morrell

Dr Preston has indicated that there are a wide variety of questions being raised in his day-to-day care of patients. It seems likely that he will be provoked to answer some of those. Only by such a critical approach to general practice will real improvements be made. Enthusiasm, however, must be tempered by judgement because it is all too easy to rush into studies in general practice without proper planning, to collect a great deal of information at considerable personal cost, only to find that the data collected are not valid and cannot be used to answer any questions. This is a most demoralizing experience and this chapter is designed to indicate some of the common pitfalls for those starting research in general practice in the hope that they may be avoided. All the pits described in this chapter have been fallen into at one time or another by the author. Learning from personal experience can be rewarding, but learning from the experience of others may be more economical and less painful

Descriptive studies in general practice.

These may be concerned with a variety of topics such as describing the way in which medical care is delivered or describing the natural history of a symptom or illness. In every case, it is essential to define clearly what is being described. If it is consultations or consultation rates, then it is important to define what is meant by a consultation and how the rates are to be calculated, i.e. to define the denominator. When describing poorly defined events, such as out-of-hours visits or repeat prescribing, this is particularly important. Where possible, definitions should be used which accord with other reported studies of the same problem so that comparison may be made.

When studying the natural history of illness in general practice there are many advantages in using, as a starting point, the symptoms presented to the doctor rather than the doctor's interpretation of these symptoms in terms of a diagnosis. This is because the problem-solving in general practice starts with the presenting symptoms, and other general practitioners will be able to identify these much more clearly than the doctors' subjective interpretation of these symptoms. In studying urinary tract infections, for instance, all patients presenting with dysuria and/or frequency of micturition may be included. Those subsequently found to have significant bacteriuria can always be separated in the analysis.

It is always important to be aware that individual general practitioners differ in the way they interpret the definitions used in a research project. If a large number of doctors are co-operating in a project it is worthwhile bringing them together to discuss, as a group, how to interpret the definitions. It can be very useful to ask them to complete the research record in response to a series of case vignettes. In this way inter-doctor variation in the way the research record will be completed can be investigated and differences ironed out in advance.

When doctors are recording not just symptoms but physical signs, more serious problems may be encountered. Roland (1983), using video recordings of examinations of a patient complaining of back pain, demonstrated how different doctors varied in the way they elicited and recorded abnormal signs and, in addition, how the patients varied in the way they responded to the doctor's examination. Watkins *et al.* (1986) have drawn attention to some of the problems of training doctors to interpret signs of respiratory illness in infants in a consistent way.

Enthusiasm to get on and launch a study may lead a researcher to ignore these very important facts concerned with definitions and minimizing inter-doctor variation in the interpretation of definitions and physical signs. If he does so, he will usually with hindsight regret it.

Complete data collection

When doctors agree to take part in a study of the natural history of symptoms or disease or in epidemiological studies concerned with the aetiology of disease, it is important that they should recruit into the study all the patients with the characteristics that are being studied. In different circumstances this may include all patients who have attended the surgery without an appointment, all patients presenting with back pain, or all patients referred to hospital. Unless all the patients with the characteristics being studied are included, it is highly likely that those excluded from the study will seriously bias the results. In studies of this type it is important to determine in advance which patients should be excluded. Once this has been agreed all other patients with the characteristics must be included. The particular study may involve the patient in answering questionnaires or undergoing a particular physical examination, and the doctor may be tempted to exclude certain patients from these procedures. When under pressure, the doctor may wish to excuse himself from undertaking extra work or may simply forget to include the patient in the study.

In the hurly-burly of general practice it can be very difficult to ensure that all patients available for study are included. It is therefore essential to build in some method to ensure that this occurs. One method is to appoint a research assistant or fieldworker to scan all the medical records after each consulting session to ensure that all the appropriate patients have been recruited. This individual may also play an important part in ensuring that the doctor has completed all the records which are demanded of the particular study. This will vary widely in different types of study. In studies in which the doctor is constrained to record certain information about every consultation on an encounter sheet, the assistant will ensure that this is done. In other studies, such as all patients suffering from dysuria, the assistant will ensure that all these patients have been included in the study and that the predetermined research record has been completed. When the doctor is involved in a randomized controlled trial, the assistant will ensure that all eligible patients have been included, that they have been properly randomized, and that the requisite records have been completed.

In planning studies in general practice it is important to bear in mind that the doctor is very often being asked to record information during a consultation. These consultations may be booked at 5–10 minute intervals. There is therefore a limit to the amount of information he can be expected to collect. Excessive demands by the researcher will almost always lead to incomplete data collection. It is also worth bearing in mind that the doctor will find it much easier to collect and record information of a type which he is accustomed to recording. It is not difficult for him to record the patient's presenting symptom, his diagnosis, or the drugs prescribed. If, however, he is asked to record details about the patient's occupation in order to allocate him to a particular social class, or to record details of housing or family structure, he is very likely to fail to complete this record. If detailed information of this type is demanded of the research, it may be better to arrange for the patient to be interviewed by a research assistant at the end of the consultation rather than to depend on the doctor collecting such information in the course of a normal consultation.

Measuring change over time

Not infrequently doctors decide to change the way in which they deliver medical care. In such a situation it is very tempting to try to measure the effect of this change. It would appear to be relatively simple to measure the changes produced by an innovation. In one experiment (Morrell and Kasap 1972) the doctors introduced an appointment system in their practice. They measured the effect of this by recording surgery consultations and home visits in two seasonally matched periods of time in successive years, one before and one after the appointment system was introduced. The results indicated a fall in demand for acute illness and a redistribution of care to the elderly in the period following the introduction of the appointment system. The researcher had assumed that by seasonally matching the periods of data collection he would avoid problems presented by different experiences in morbidity. Studies of sickness absence and mortality data in the years under study, however, proved this assumption to be wrong and the findings of the study must be suspect. If a nearby practice had been asked to record information over the same periods and to act as a control, the value of the study would have been enhanced.

Measuring changes over time is subject to a variety of hazards. There are the changes in morbidity experienced in different seasons and in different years (in some practices there are changes in the population in winter and summer), there are changes in statutory regulations such as prescription charges, sickness absence certification, etc. There are, in addition, the immediate changes within a practice in terms of the personnel working in the practice or the attached community nurses and health visitors. All of these can affect the delivery of medical care, and it is often difficult to determine whether the particular experiment in the practice has or has not influenced the uptake or distribution of care. Ideally a random sample in the practice would be exposed to the new method of delivering care, but this is rarely possible because of contamination of the control group and major difficulties in practice management and the relationship between doctors and patients. This is a classical example of the conflict between the epidemiological ideal and what is practical in the real world of the general practice.

Cohort studies

Studying a cohort of patients in general practice over a period of years can offer unique opportunities to describe the natural history of disease. Such studies may be concerned with particular age groups in the practice or with cohorts of patients suffering from particular symptoms or diseases. The main difficulty presented in this type of study arises from the mobility of the individuals in the cohort. In some general practices up to 20 per cent of the patients may migrate out of the practice each year. Before undertaking such a study, it is therefore important to obtain some estimate of migration rates. These estimates should be age-specific because in some practices certain age groups may be highly mobile while others are relatively stable. In addition it is helpful to get some estimate of where patients migrate to. In Inner London, for instance, many patients may change their address within the practice or to relatively close geographical locations. In other situations patients may migrate right across the country.

In studies in which patients will be followed up for just one or two years, migration may not be a serious problem, but in longer term studies an important proportion of the population may be lost to follow-up. In tracing patients who have migrated, Family Practitioner Committees (FPCs) may be helpful in providing the name of the new doctor with whom the patient has registered, and council housing departments can sometimes provide useful information. In some cohort studies the researcher has sent birthday cards to the members of the cohort with a 'tear-off' slip to notify change of address. In studies in the elderly, death, which can be an important outcome variable, may lead to loss of patients from follow-up. At a price, death certification data can be obtained from Somerset House. In developing cohort studies, it is important to realize that follow-up of the cohort is likely to be time-consuming and expensive and it is important to allow for this in making grant applications.

Controlled trials

In developing randomized controlled trials of treatment in general practice, there are a variety of ways of allocating patients to the active and placebo groups. This may be done by the use of random numbers. This can be applied in a practice in which each patient has a unique serial number and sometimes randomization is delegated to a receptionist who has a bunch of envelopes containing alternative treatments stored in random order. Alternatively the doctor may allocate the treatment based on the patient's date of birth in the month. Before random allocation of treatments can occur, however, the doctor must obtain the patient's consent to enter the trial. In general practice this can produce some problems. The general practitioner has a close and continuing relationship with his patients. He almost inevitably has a biased opinion about the value and side-effects of the alternative treatments being prescribed. As a result, he may consciously or subconsciously exclude individual patients from the trial. Most randomized controlled trials of treatments state clearly which patients should be excluded, but it is not unknown to find that these exclusion criteria can be interpreted in a variety of ways. If valid results are to be obtained, very careful supervision of controlled trials is required, and there must be adequate opportunity for meeting those doctors involved to discuss and resolve difficulties.

A further problem occurs in measuring the results of the treatment under trial. Very few doctors can take a totally objective view of the outcome of the trial, particularly when their patients are involved. In this situation it may be helpful to have a totally unbiased research assistant responsible for recording the outcome measures. Many trials are described as double-blind, but it can be extremely difficult to keep the doctor blind. An example of this occurred in trials of diuretics in the management of hypertension. The doctor was unaware of the treatment his patient was receiving until the quarterly reports on the patient's serum potassium levels and urate levels made it very obvious which patients were receiving diuretics.

Measuring patient satisfaction

This is a recurring problem in studies carried out in general practice. It is apparent that patients have difficulty in expressing dissatisfaction with their doctor particularly when questioned about this on his consulting premises. General questions about satisfaction may produce useful results, but questions directed to measure satisfaction with individual aspects of the issue being studied may be more useful. Questions designed to measure satisfaction and administered in the patient's home by someone explicitly unconnected with the practice and some days after the consultation may provide a more objective measure, but they are expensive to carry out and are dependent on the patient's recall of the consultation.

Check-list of problems

In designing a study in general practice it may be helpful to have a check-list of the sort of problems which may be encountered. The following have been drawn up as a result of the author's experience:

Sampling	Is it a random sample of the population? Is it permissible to replace non-respondents (or will it bias the results)? If a selected sample, how is it defined? How mobile is the population?
Data collection	Do methods ensure that data will be complete? How will you handle missing data? If follow-up is necessary, how is it ensured? Are you sure all definitions are agreed? If 'diagnosis' is used, has it been defined? Have you 'piloted' your methods of data collection?
Interpreting results	Have you excluded or measured bias in outcome measures? Is population subject to changes over time? Is practice subject to changes over time? What other factors could explain your results?

Writing a research protocol

Perhaps the most important pit into which researchers in general practice fall is starting a research project without drawing up a detailed protocol in advance, describing each step of the study. To a general practitioner who is doing his first small research project it may seem to be unnecessarily pedantic to write down every detail about sampling techniques, the definitions applied, and the methods of data collection and processing. If this is not done, however, serious mistakes can be made. In addition, a protocol is essential if an application is to be made for research funding. A research protocol should be seen as similar to an architect's plans for building a house. It describes the overall objective, the actions which will be taken at each stage in creating the project, and the resources which will be necessary to bring the project to a successful conclusion. Some of the important features of a research protocol may be summarized, as follows:

Introduction—This should describe the need for the study. It should contain references to other studies which illustrate the relevance of the project.

Aim of study. This should state briefly but very clearly what the study is designed to achieve.

Statement of problems and overall plan of study. This should describe in general terms how you plan to undertake the study. It should be a summary of the detailed method which then follows.

Details of method. In this section the exact procedures to be undertaken in the study should be described in detail. It should demonstrate that the proposal is practical and that you have allowed for all the likely problems to be encountered. It should describe in detail the population to be studied, methods of sampling, definitions to be used, questionnaires or laboratory methods to be employed, etc. It should describe in detail how the data will be collected, verified, and analysed. A flow diagram may be helpful at this stage.

Procedures during study. This should detail the timetable of the study, indicating what is to be achieved at each stage.

Evaluation and interpretation. This should describe in detail how you intend to analyse the data to answer the main questions posed by the study.

Application of findings. This should spell out how your findings may be applied and how they may be expected to improve knowledge or care.

Proposed schedule. This should include details of the staff and resources required at each stage of the study.

Budget. Draw up the expected costs. This should include staff, and allow for superannuation and expected pay rises, travel, durable and non-durable equipment, not forgetting resources for data analysis, secretarial services, and stationary.

A series of appendices may be attached, including, for instance, forms to be used in recording data, questionnaires, and details of data processing.

Obtaining support

Many research projects in general practice founder because they are not properly planned and resourced. In almost all studies which are designed to answer a specific question or test a hypothesis, a statistician should be consulted early in the planning stage. In purely descriptive studies or studies concerned with developing new methods of care the help of a statistician will also be invaluable if there is an element of evaluation in the work. Do not expect a statistician to analyse your data unless he has been involved in the design stage.

Make sure you have adequate resources to undertake the project. Additional clerical help can make the difference between success and failure. If the study is concerned with improving patient care in your practice, then it is perfectly legitimate to employ an extra clerical worker to help with data collection and supervision and to charge 70 per cent of the salary to the FPC. If extra funding is needed make sure that this covers all aspects of the study, including, in particular, travel and data processing. In seeking research funding try to identify the research interests of the funding bodies and apply to those most in sympathy with your work.

Always do a pilot study

Last, but by no means least, always carry out a pilot study before embarking on a major research project. This will reveal all the likely problems to be encountered in the main study. It should be as meticulously planned as the main study and designed to reveal weaknesses in such aspects of the study as sampling methods, data collection, use of definitions, and testing and validating questionnaires. The time spent on a pilot study will never be wasted. No one has ever regretted doing a pilot study, but many have learned too late that the failure to pilot their research methods has led to untold anguish because of unpredictable problems which have rendered their research valueless.

CONCLUSION

There are many pitfalls awaiting the general practitioner who wishes to carry out research in his practice. Some of these are related to the fact that few general practitioners have been taught how to undertake a research project. Others are related to the fact that general practitioners have a very special relationship with their patients, often spanning years of repeated contact which offers unique opportunities but carries with it serious responsibilities. Others are due to the fact that the average consultation in general practice lasts just a few minutes and collecting complex research data is difficult in this setting. These are some of the reasons why good research based on valid data are relatively uncommon in general practice. At the same time it must be stressed that there are important areas of medical care concerned with the natural history of disease, the delivery of care, and the aetiology of disease which can only be conducted in general practice. From this it must be concluded that general practitioner researchers of the future, if they are to attain their full potential, must be fully aware of the epidemiological principles which underpin good research, but must also learn how to apply these in the setting in which they work.

REFERENCES

Morrell, D. C. and Kasap. H. (1972). The effect of an appointment system on demand for medical care. *International Journal of Epidemiology* **1,** 143–51.

Roland, M. O. (1983). Videotape as a research tool. *Journal of the Royal College of General Practitioners* **33,** 300–1.

Watkins, C. J., Sittampalam, Y., Morrell, D. C., Leader, S., and Tritton, E. (1986). Patterns of respiratory illness in the first year of life. *British Medical Journal* **293,** 794–6.

Index